NEUROLOGICAL EXAMINATION

MADE EASY

GERAINT FULLER MD FRCP

Consultant Neurologist
Gloucester Royal Hospital
Gloucester
UK

FIFTH EDITION

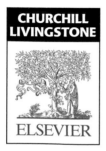
CHURCHILL
LIVINGSTONE

ELSEVIER

Edinburgh London New York Oxford Philadelphia St Louis Sydney Toronto 2013

CHURCHILL
LIVINGSTONE
ELSEVIER

First edition 1993
Second edition 1999
Third edition 2004
Fourth edition 2008

ISBN 978-0-7020-5177-7
International ISBN 978-0-7020-5178-4

British Library Cataloguing in Publication Data
A catalogue record for this book is available from the British Library

Library of Congress Cataloging in Publication Data
A catalog record for this book is available from the Library of Congress

Notices
Knowledge and best practice in this field are constantly changing. As new research and experience broaden our understanding, changes in research methods, professional practices, or medical treatment may become necessary.

Practitioners and researchers must always rely on their own experience and knowledge in evaluating and using any information, methods, compounds, or experiments described herein. In using such information or methods they should be mindful of their own safety and the safety of others, including parties for whom they have a professional responsibility.

With respect to any drug or pharmaceutical products identified, readers are advised to check the most current information provided (i) on procedures featured or (ii) by the manufacturer of each product to be administered, to verify the recommended dose or formula, the method and duration of administration, and contraindications. It is the responsibility of practitioners, relying on their own experience and knowledge of their patients, to make diagnoses, to determine dosages and the best treatment for each individual patient, and to take all appropriate safety precautions.

To the fullest extent of the law, neither the Publisher nor the authors, contributors, or editors, assume any liability for any injury and/or damage to persons or property as a matter of products liability, negligence or otherwise, or from any use or operation of any methods, products, instructions, or ideas contained in the material herein.

ELSEVIER   your source for books,
journals and multimedia
in the health sciences

www.elsevierhealth.com

    Working together
to grow libraries in
developing countries

www.elsevier.com • www.bookaid.org

The
publisher's
policy is to use
**paper manufactured
from sustainable forests**

Printed in China

CONTENTS

ACKNOWLEDGEMENTS

I would like to thank all my teachers, particularly Dr Roberto Guiloff, who introduced me to neurology. I am grateful to the many medical students at Charing Cross and Westminster Medical School who have acted as guinea pigs in the preparation of the previous editions of this book and to the colleagues who have kindly commented on the text. I am also most appreciative of all the constructive comments made about the earlier editions of the book by students, mainly from Bristol University, junior doctors and colleagues, and particularly the neurologists involved in its translation. For this latest edition I am grateful to Mark Wiles, Robin Howard and Rhys Thomas for their thoughtful comments and to Peter Scanlon for help with fundal photographs.

In learning to be a clinical neurologist and in writing this book, I am indebted to a wide range of textbooks and scientific papers that are too many to mention.

This book is dedicated to Cherith.

INTRODUCTION

Many medical students and junior doctors think that neurological examination is extremely complicated and difficult.

This is because:

- they find it hard to remember what to do
- they are not sure what they are looking for
- they do not know how to describe what they find.

The aim of this book is to provide a simple framework to allow a medical student or junior doctor to perform a straightforward neurological examination. It explains what to do and points out common problems and mistakes. This book cannot replace conventional bedside teaching and clinical experience.

Inevitably, when trying to simplify the range of neurological findings and their interpretation, not all possible situations can be anticipated. This book has been designed to try to accommodate most common situations and tries to warn of common pitfalls; there will be some occasions where incorrect conclusions will be reached.

How to use this book

This book concentrates on how to perform the neurological part of a physical examination. Each chapter starts with a brief background and relevant information. This is followed by a section telling you 'What to do', both in a straightforward case and in the presence of abnormalities. The abnormalities that can be found are then described in the 'What you find' section, and finally the 'What it means' section provides an interpretation of the findings and suggests potential pathologies.

It is important to understand that the neurological examination can be used as:

- a screening test
- an investigative tool.

It is used as a screening test when you examine a patient in whom you expect to find no neurological abnormalities: for example, a patient with a non-neurological disease or a patient with a neurological illness not normally associated with physical abnormalities, such as migraine or epilepsy. Neurological examination is used as an investigative tool in patients when a neurological abnormality is found on screening, or when an abnormality can be expected from the history. The aim of examination is to determine whether there is an abnormality, determining its nature and extent and seeking associated abnormalities.

There is no ideal neurological examination technique. The methods of neurological examination have evolved gradually. There are conventional ways to perform an examination, a conventional order of examination and conventional ways to elicit particular signs. Most neurologists have developed their own system for examination, a variation on the conventional techniques. In this book, one such variation is presented and aims to provide a skeleton for students to flesh out with their own personal variations.

In this book, each part of the examination is dealt with separately. This is to allow description and understanding of abnormalities in each part of the examination. However, these parts need to be considered together in evaluating a patient as a whole. Thus, the findings in total need to be synthesised.

The synthesis of the examination findings should be as described below.

1. Anatomical
Can the findings be explained by:

- one lesion
- multiple lesions
- a diffuse process?

What level/levels of the nervous systems is/are affected (Fig. 0.1)?

2. Syndromal
Do the clinical findings combine to form a recognisable clinical syndrome: for example, parkinsonism, motor neurone disease, multiple sclerosis?

3. Aetiological
Once you have come to an anatomical or syndromal synthesis, consider what pathological processes could have caused this:

- genetic
- congenital
- infectious
- inflammatory
- neoplastic
- degenerative
- traumatic
- metabolic and toxic
- paroxysmal (including migraine and epilepsy)
- endocrine
- vascular?

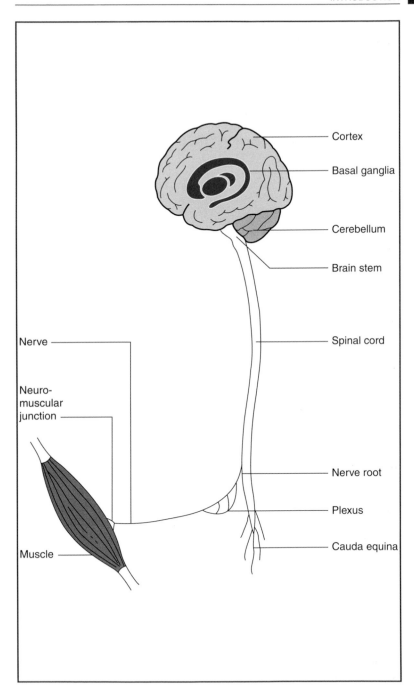

Figure 0.1
The levels of the nervous system

The interpretation of the neurological history and the synthesis of the neurological examination require experience and background knowledge. This book will not be able to provide these. However, using this book you should be able to describe, using appropriate terms, most of the common neurological abnormalities and you will begin to be able to synthesise and interpret them.

Throughout the book, the patient and examiner are presumed to be male, to avoid the awkward use of he/she.

Cranial nerves will be referred to by their name, or by their number in roman numerals.

Neurological terms

Neurological terms have evolved and some terms may be used in different ways by different neurologists.

Here are some terms used to describe pathologies at different levels of the nervous system.

-opathy: suffix indicating abnormality at the level of the nervous system indicated in the prefix; see *encephalopathy* below. Cf. *-itis*.
-itis: suffix indicating inflammation of the level of the nervous system indicated in the prefix; see *myelitis* below.
Encephalopathy: abnormality of the brain. May be refined by adjectives such as *focal* or *diffuse*, or *metabolic* or *toxic*.
Encephalitis: inflammation of the brain. May be refined by adjectives such as *focal* or *diffuse*. May be combined with other terms to indicate associated disease, e.g. *meningo-encephalitis=meningitis* and *encephalitis*.
Meningitis: inflammation of the meninges.
Myelopathy: abnormality of the spinal cord. Refined by terms indicating aetiology, e.g. *radiation, compressive*.
Myelitis: inflammation of the spinal cord.
Radiculopathy: abnormality of a nerve root.
Plexopathy: abnormality of nerve plexus (brachial or lumbar).
Peripheral neuropathy: abnormality of peripheral nerves. Usually refined using adjectives such as *diffuse/multifocal, sensory/sensorimotor/motor* and *acute/chronic*.
Polyradiculopathy: abnormality of many nerve roots. Usually reserved for proximal nerve damage and to contrast this with length-dependent nerve damage.
Polyneuropathy: similar term to peripheral neuropathy, but may be used to contrast with *polyradiculopathy*.
Mononeuropathy: abnormality of a single nerve.
Myopathy: abnormality of muscle.
Myositis: inflammatory disorder of muscle.
Functional: term used in two ways: (1) non-structural pathology—an abnormality of function: for example, migraine; (2) as a term for psychiatrically induced neurological abnormalities including, for example, hysterical conversion.

1

HISTORY AND EXAMINATION

HISTORY

The history is the most important part of the neurological evaluation. Just as detectives gain most information about the identity of a criminal from witnesses rather than from the examination of the scene of the crime, neurologists learn most about the likely pathology from the history rather than the examination.

The general approach to the history is common to all complaints. Which parts of the history prove to be most important will obviously vary according to the particular complaint. An outline for approaching the history is given below. The history is usually presented in a conventional way (below) so that doctors being informed of or reading the history know what they going to be told about next. Everyone develops their own way of taking a history and doctors often adapt the way they do it depending on the clinical problem facing them. This section is organised according to the usual way in which a history is presented—recognising that sometimes elements of the history can be obtained in a different order.

Many neurologists would regard history taking, rather than neurological examination, as their special skill (though you obviously need both). This indicates the importance attached to history taking within neurology, and reflects that it is an active process, requiring listening, thinking and reflective questioning rather than simply passive note taking. There is now evidence that it is not just what the patient says, but the way he says it that can be diagnostically useful (for example in the diagnosis of non-epileptic attack disorder).

The neurological history

- Age, sex, handedness, occupation
- History of present complaint
- Neurological screening questions
- Past medical history
- Drug history
- Family history
- Social history.

Basic background information

Establish some basic background information initially—the age, sex, handedness and occupation (or previous occupation) of the patient.

Handedness is important. The left hemisphere contains language in almost all right-handed individuals, and in 70% of patients who are left-handed or ambidextrous.

Present complaint

Start with an open question such as 'Tell me all about it from the very beginning' or 'What has been happening?'. Try to let patients tell their story in their own words with minimum interruption. The patient may need to be encouraged to start from the beginning. Often patients want to tell you what is happening now. You will find this easier to understand if you know what events led up to the current situation.

Whilst listening to their story, try to determine (Fig. 1.1):

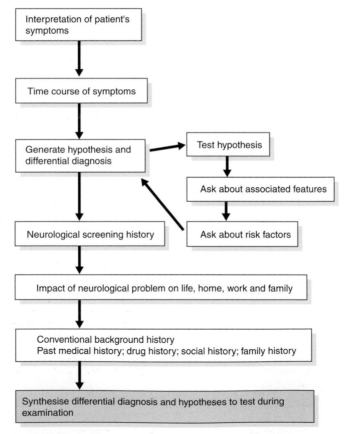

Figure 1.1
Flow chart: the present complaint

- *The nature of the complaint.* Make sure you have understood what the patient is describing. For example, dizziness may mean vertigo (the true sensation of spinning) or lightheadedness or a swimming sensation in the head. When a patient says his vision is blurred, he may mean it is double. A patient with weakness but no altered sensation may refer to his limb as numb.

 TIP   It is better to get an exact description for specific events, particularly the first, last and most severe events, rather than an abstracted summary of a typical event.

- *The time course.* This tells you about the tempo of the pathology (Table 1.1 and Fig. 1.2).
  - The onset: How did it come on? Suddenly, over a few seconds, a few minutes, hours, days, weeks or months?
  - Progression: Is it continuous or intermittent? Has it improved, stabilised or progressed (gradually or in a stepwise fashion)? When describing the progression, use a functional gauge where possible: for example, the ability to run, walk, using one stick, walking with a frame or walker.
  - The pattern: If intermittent, what was its duration and what was its frequency?

Table 1.1
Some illustrations of how time course indicates pathology

Time course	Pathological process
A 50-year-old man with complete visual loss in his right eye	
Came on suddenly and lasted 1 minute	Vascular: impaired blood flow to the retina; 'amaurosis fugax'
Came on over 10 minutes and lasted 20 minutes	Migrainous
Came on over 4 days and then improved over 6 weeks	Inflammatory; inflammation in the optic nerve; 'optic neuritis'
Progressed over 3 months	Optic nerve compression; possibly from a meningioma
A 65-year-old woman with left-sided face, arm and leg weakness	
Came on suddenly and lasted 10 minutes	Vascular: transient ischaemic attack
Came on over 10 minutes and persists several days later	Vascular: stroke
Came on over 4 weeks	Consider subdural tumour
Came on over 4 months	Likely to be tumour
Has been there since childhood	Congenital

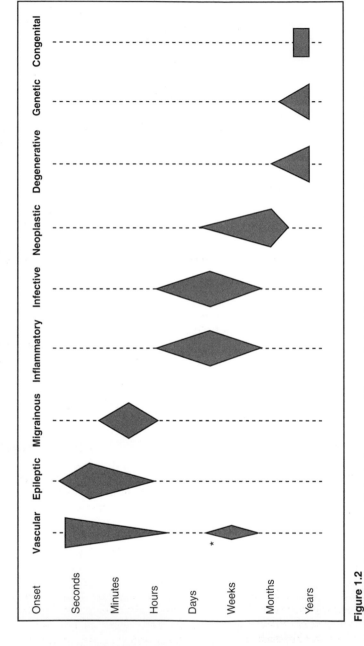

Figure 1.2
The tempo of different pathological processes. The onset of metabolic and endocrinological problems relates to the rate of onset of the metabolic or endocrine problem. *Late vascular problems from chronic subdural haematoma

TIP It can be useful to summarise the history, thinking about how you would describe the time course, as the terms used can point towards the relevant underlying pathological process. For example: *sudden onset or acute* suggests vascular; *subacute* suggests inflammation, infection or neoplasia; *progressive* suggests neoplasia or degenerative; *stepwise or stuttering* suggests vascular or inflammation; *relapsing–remitting* suggests inflammation.

 TIP Remember: when a patient cannot report all events himself or cannot give a history adequately for another reason such as a speech problem, it is essential to get the history from others if at all possible, such as relatives, friends or even passers-by.
   If you cannot see them in person – call them on the telephone!

Also determine:

- *Precipitating or relieving factors.* Remember that a spontaneously reported symptom is much more significant than one obtained on direct questioning. For example, patients rarely volunteer that their headaches get worse on coughing or sneezing, and when they do it suggests raised intracranial pressure. In contrast, many patients with tension-type headaches and migraine will say their headaches get worse in these situations if directly asked about them.
- *Previous treatments and investigations.* Prior treatments may have helped or have produced adverse effects. This information may help in planning future treatments.
- *The current neurological state.* What can the patient do now? Determine current abilities in relation to normal everyday activities. Clearly, this needs to be done differently for different types of problem we consider in relation to work and mobility (can he walk normally or what is the level of impairment?), and ability to eat, wash and go to the toilet.
- *Hypothesis generation and testing.* Whilst listening, think about what might be causing the patient's problems. This may suggest associated problems or precipitating factors that would be worth exploring. For example, if a patient's history makes you wonder whether he has Parkinson's disease, ask about his handwriting—something you would probably not talk about with most patients.
- *Screening for other neurological symptoms.* Determine whether the patient has had any headaches, fits, faints, blackouts, episodes of numbness, tingling or weakness, any sphincter disturbance (urinary or faecal incontinence, urinary retention and constipation) or visual symptoms, including double vision, blurred vision or loss of sight. This is unlikely to provide any surprises if hypothesis testing has been successful.

COMMON MISTAKES

- Patients frequently want to tell you about the doctors they have seen before and what these doctors have done and said, rather than describing what has been happening to them personally. This is usually misleading and must be regarded with caution. If this information would be useful to you, it is better obtained directly from the doctors concerned. Most patients can be redirected to give their history rather than the history of their medical contacts.
- You interrupt the story with a list of questions. If uninterrupted, patients usually only talk for 1–2 minutes before stopping. Listen first, then clarify what you do not understand later.
- The history just does not seem to make sense. This tends to happen in patients with speech, memory or concentration difficulties and in those with non-organic disease. Think of aphasia, depression, dementia and hysteria.

 TIP   It is often useful to summarise the essential points of the history to the patient—to make sure that you have understood them correctly. This is called 'chunking and checking'.

Conventional history

Past medical history

This is important to help understand the aetiology or discover conditions associated with neurological conditions. For example, a history of hypertension is important in patients with stroke; a history of diabetes in patients with peripheral neuropathy; and a history of previous cancer surgery in patients with focal cerebral abnormalities suggesting possible metastases.

It is always useful to consider the basis for any diagnosis given by the patient. For example, a patient with a past medical history that starts with 'known epilepsy' may not in fact have epilepsy; once the diagnosis is accepted, it is rarely questioned and patients may be treated inappropriately.

Drug history

It is essential to check what prescribed drugs and over-the-counter medicines are being taken. This can act as a reminder of the conditions the patient may have forgotten (hypertension and asthma). Drugs can also cause neurological problems—it is often worth checking their adverse effects.

N.B. Many women do not think of the oral contraceptive as a drug and need to be asked about it specifically.

Family history
Many neurological problems have a genetic basis, so a detailed family history is often very important in making the diagnosis. Even if no one in the family is identified with a potentially relevant neurological problem, information about the family is helpful. For example, think about what a 'negative' family history means in:

- a patient with no siblings whose parents, both only children, died at a young age from an unrelated problem (for example, trauma)
- a patient with seven living older siblings and living parents (each of whom has four younger living siblings).

The former might well have a familial problem though the family history is uninformative; the latter would be very unlikely to have an inherited problem.

In some circumstances, patients can be reluctant to tell you about certain inherited problems: for example, Huntington's disease. On other occasions, other family members can be very mildly affected; for example, in the hereditary motor and sensory neuropathies, some family members will simply be aware that they have high arched feet, so this needs to be actively sought if it is likely to be relevant.

Social history
Neurological patients frequently have significant disability. For these patients, the environment in which they normally live, their financial circumstances, their family and carers in the community are all very important to their current and future care.

Toxin exposure
It is important to establish any exposure to toxins, including in this category both tobacco and alcohol, as well as industrial neurotoxins.

Systemic inquiry
Systemic inquiry may reveal clues that general medical disease may be presenting with neurological manifestations. For example, a patient with atherosclerosis may have angina and intermittent claudication as well as symptoms of cerebrovascular disease.

Patient's perception of illness
Ask patients what they think is wrong with them. This is useful when you discuss the diagnosis with them. If they turn out to be right, you know they have already thought about the possibility. If they have

something else, it is also helpful to explain why they do not have what they suggested and probably are particularly concerned about. For example, if they have migraine but were concerned that they had a brain tumour, it is helpful to discuss this differential diagnosis specifically.

Anything else?

Always include an open question towards the end of the history— 'Is there anything else you wanted to tell me about?'—to make sure patients have had the chance to tell you everything they wanted to.

Synthesis of history and differential diagnosis

It is useful to summarise the history before moving on to the examination—in your own mind at least—and try to come to a differential diagnosis. The type of differential diagnosis will vary according to the patient—some examples:

- In a patient with a history of wrist drop, your main question may be whether this is a radial nerve palsy, C7 radiculopathy or something else.
- In a patient with right-sided slowness, you might wonder whether what they have is a movement disorder, such as Parkinson's disease, or an upper motor neurone weakness.

If you think about the differential at this stage, you can then be sure to use the examination to try to come to a diagnosis.

So, think about the differential diagnosis generated from the history. Think what might be found on examination in these circumstances and ensure you focus on these possibilities during your examination.

In summary, think about the history.

GENERAL EXAMINATION

General examination may yield important clues as to the diagnosis of neurological disease. Examination may find systemic disease with neurological complications (Fig. 1.3 and Table 1.2).

A full general examination is therefore important in assessing a patient with neurological disease. The features that need to be particularly looked for in an unconscious patient are dealt with in Chapter 27.

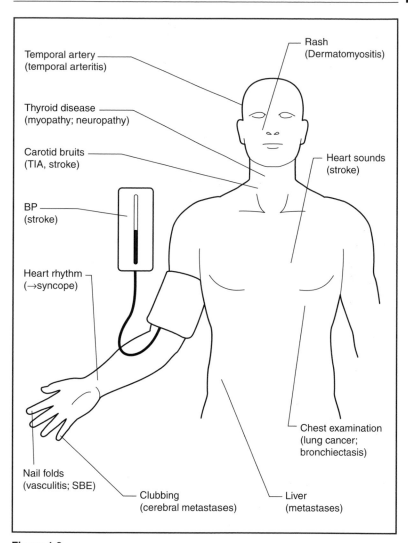

Figure 1.3
General examination of neurological relevance. (SBE = subacute bacterial
endocarditis; TIA = transient ischaemic attack)

Table 1.2
Examination findings in systemic disease with neurological complications

Disease	Sign	Neurological condition
Degenerative diseases		
Atherosclerosis	Carotid bruit	Stroke
Valvular heart disease	Murmur	Stroke
Inflammatory disease		
Rheumatoid arthritis	Arthritis and rheumatoid nodules	Neuropathies Cervical cord compression
Endocrine disease		
Hypothyroidism	Abnormal facies, skin, hair	Cerebellar syndrome Myopathy
Diabetes	Retinal changes Injection marks	Neuropathy
Neoplasia		
Lung cancer	Pleural effusion	Cerebral metastases
Breast cancer	Breast mass	Cerebral metastases
Dermatological disease		
Dermatomyositis	Heliotrope rash	Dermatomyositis

2

SPEECH

BACKGROUND

Abnormalities of speech need to be considered first, as these may interfere with your history taking and subsequent ability to assess other aspects of higher function and perform the rest of the examination.

Abnormalities of speech can reflect abnormalities anywhere along the following chain shown.

PROCESS	ABNORMALITY
Hearing	Deafness
Understanding	
Thought and word finding }	Aphasia
Voice production	Dysphonia
Articulation	Dysarthria

Problems with deafness are dealt with in Chapter 12.

1. Aphasia

In this book, the term aphasia will be used to refer to all disorders of understanding, thought and word finding. Dysphasia is a term used by some to indicate a disorder of speech, reserving aphasia to mean absence of speech.

Aphasia has been classified in a number of ways and each new classification has brought some new terminology. There are therefore a number of terms that refer to broadly similar problems:

- Broca's aphasia = expressive aphasia = motor aphasia
- Wernicke's aphasia = receptive aphasia = sensory aphasia
- nominal aphasia = anomic aphasia.

Most of these systems have evolved from a simple model of aphasia (Fig. 2.1). In this model, sounds are recognised as language in Wernicke's area, which is then connected to a 'concept area' where

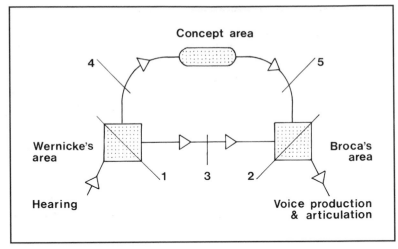

Figure 2.1
Simple model of speech understanding and output

the meaning of the words is understood. The 'concept area' is connected to Broca's area, where speech output is generated. Wernicke's area is also connected directly to Broca's area by the arcuate fasciculus. These areas are in the dominant hemisphere and are described later. The left hemisphere is dominant in right-handed patients and some left-handed patients, and the right hemisphere is dominant in some left-handed patients.

The following patterns of aphasia can be recognised and are associated with lesions at the sites as numbered on the figure:

1. **Wernicke's aphasia**—poor comprehension; fluent but often meaningless (as it cannot be internally checked) speech; no repetition
2. **Broca's aphasia**—preserved comprehension; non-fluent speech; no repetition
3. **Conductive aphasia**—loss of repetition with preserved comprehension and output
4. **Transcortical sensory aphasia**—as in (1) but with preserved repetition
5. **Transcortical motor aphasia**—as in (2) but with preserved repetition

Reading and writing are further aspects of language. These can also be included in models such as the one above. Not surprisingly, the models become quite complicated!

2. Dysphonia

This is a disturbance of voice production and may reflect either local vocal cord pathology (such as laryngitis), an abnormality of the nerve supply via the vagus, or occasionally a psychological disturbance.

3. Dysarthria

Voice production requires coordination of breathing, vocal cords, larynx, palate, tongue and lips. Dysarthria can therefore reflect difficulties at different levels.

Lesions of upper motor neurone type, of the extrapyramidal system (such as Parkinson's disease) and cerebellar lesions disturb the integration of processes of speech production and tend to disturb the rhythm of speech.

Lesions of one or several of the cranial nerves tend to produce characteristic distortion of certain parts of speech but the rhythm is normal.

1. APHASIA

WHAT TO DO

Speech abnormalities may hinder or prevent taking a history from the patient. If so, **take the history from relatives or friends.**

Establish if the patient is **right- or left-handed.**
Discover the patient's **first language.**

Assess understanding

Ask the patient a simple question:

• What is your name and address?
• What is/was your job? Explain exactly what you do.
• Where do you come from?

If he does not appear to understand:

• Repeat louder.

Test understanding

• Ask questions with **yes/no answers:**
  – e.g. 'Is this a pen?' (showing something else, then a pen).
• Give a simple command:
  – e.g. 'Open your mouth' or 'With your right hand touch your nose.'
• If successful, try more complicated commands:
  – e.g. 'With your right hand touch your nose and then your left ear.'
• Define how much is understood.

 TIP Remember: if patients are weak, they may not be able to perform simple tasks.

Assess spontaneous speech

If the patient does appear to understand but is unable to speak:

- Ask if he has difficulty in finding the right words. This often brings a nod and a smile, indicating pleasure that you understand the problem.
- If the problem is less severe, he may be able to tell you his name and address slowly.

Ask further questions

Enquire, for example, about the patient's job or how the problem started.

- Is speech fluent?
- Does he use words correctly?
- Does he use the **wrong word** (*paraphasia*) or is it **meaningless jargon** (sometimes called *jargon aphasia*)?

Assess word-finding ability and naming

- Ask the patient to name all the animals he can think of (normal= 18–22 in 1 minute).
- Ask him to give all the words he can think of beginning with a particular letter, usually 'f' or 's' (abnormal=less than 12 in 1 minute for each letter).

These are tests of word finding. The test can be quantified by counting the number of objects within a standard time.

- Ask him to name familiar objects that are to hand, e.g. a watch, watch strap, buckle, shirt, tie, buttons. Start with easily named objects and later ask about less frequently used objects that will be more difficult.

Assess repetition

- Ask the patient to repeat a simple phrase, e.g. 'The sun is shining', and then increasingly complicated phrases.

Assess severity of impairment of speech

- Is the aphasia socially incapacitating?

Further tests

Test reading and writing

- Check there is no visual impairment and that usual reading glasses are used.
- Ask the patient to:
  - read a sentence
  - obey a written command, e.g. 'Close your eyes'
  - write a sentence (check there is no motor disability to prevent this).
- Impaired reading=*dyslexia*. Impaired writing=*dysgraphia*.

TIP   If there are difficulties, check the patient is normally
able to read and write.

WHAT YOU FIND

See Figure 2.2.

Before continuing your examination, describe your findings: for
example, 'This man has a socially incapacitating non-fluent global
aphasia which is predominantly expressive, with paraphasia and impaired repetition. There is associated dyslexia and dysgraphia.'

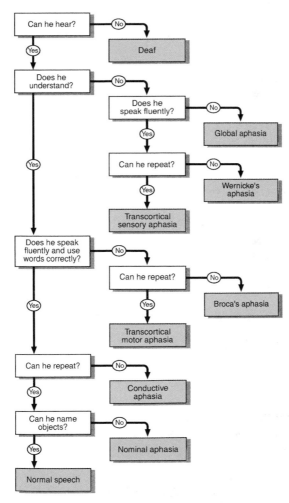

Figure 2.2
Flow chart: aphasia

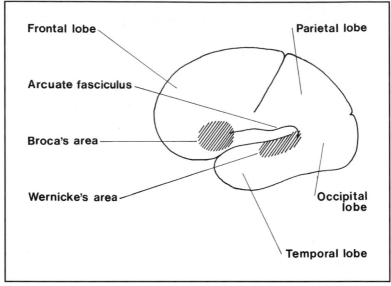

Figure 2.3
Diagram of the brain showing the location of Broca's and Wernicke's areas

WHAT IT MEANS

- **Aphasia**: lesion in the *dominant* (usually left) hemisphere.
- **Global aphasia**: lesion in the *dominant* hemisphere affecting both Wernicke's and Broca's areas (Fig. 2.3).
- **Wernicke's aphasia**: lesion in *Wernicke's area* (supramarginal gyrus of the parietal lobe and upper part of the temporal lobe). May be associated with field defect.
- **Broca's aphasia**: lesion in *Broca's area* (inferior frontal gyrus). May be associated with a hemiplegia.
- **Conductive aphasia**: lesion in *arcuate fasciculus*.
- **Transcortical sensory aphasia**: lesion in the *posterior parieto-occipital region*.
- **Transcortical motor aphasia**: incomplete lesion in *Broca's area*.
- **Nominal aphasia**: lesion in the *angular gyrus*.

Common causes are given on page 32 under Focal Deficits.

2. DYSPHONIA

WHAT TO DO

If the patient is able to give his name and address but is unable to produce a normal volume of sound or speaks in a whisper, this is *dysphonia*.

- **Ask the patient to cough.** Listen to the quality of the cough.
- **Ask the patient to say a sustained 'eeeeee'.** Does it fatigue?

WHAT YOU FIND AND WHAT IT MEANS

- Normal cough: the motor supply to the vocal cords is intact.
- Dysphonia + normal cough: local laryngeal problems or hysteria.
- Cough lacks explosive start—a bovine cough: vocal cord palsy.
- The note cannot be sustained and fatigues: consider myasthenia.

3. DYSARTHRIA

WHAT TO DO

If the patient is able to give his name and address but the words are not formed properly, he has *dysarthria* (Fig. 2.4).

Ask the patient to repeat difficult phrases, e.g. 'Peter Piper picked a peck of pickled pepper' or 'The Leith policeman dismisseth us'. Two very useful phrases are:

- 'yellow lorry': tests lingual (tongue) sounds
- 'baby hippopotamus': tests labial (lip) sounds.

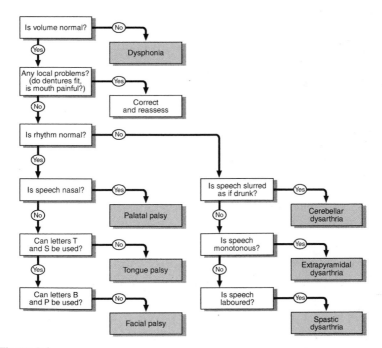

Figure 2.4
Flow chart: dysarthria

Listen carefully for:

- the rhythm of the speech
- slurred words
- which sounds cause the greatest difficulty.

WHAT YOU FIND

Types of dysarthria

With abnormal rhythm

- **Spastic**: slurred, slowed and laboured; the patient hardly opens the mouth, as if trying to speak from the back of the mouth.
- **Extrapyramidal**: monotonous, without rhythm, sentences suddenly start and stop.
- **Cerebellar**: slurred as if drunk, disjointed rhythm sometimes with scanning speech (equal emphasis on each syllable).

With normal rhythm

- Lower motor neurone:
  - *Palatal*: nasal speech, as with a bad cold
  - *Tongue*: distorted speech, especially letters t, s and d
  - *Facial*: difficulty with b, p, m and w, the sounds avoided by ventriloquists.
- Myasthenic:
  - Muscle fatigability is demonstrated by making the patient count.
  - Observe for the development of dysphonia or a lower motor neurone pattern of dysarthria. (N.B. Myasthenia gravis is a failure of neuromuscular transmission.)

Before continuing your examination, describe your findings.

WHAT IT MEANS

- **Spastic dysarthria**: bilateral upper motor neurone weakness. *Causes*: pseudobulbar palsy (diffuse cerebrovascular disease), motor neurone disease.
- **Extrapyramidal dysarthria**. *Common cause*: parkinsonism.
- **Cerebellar dysarthria.** *Common causes*: alcohol intoxication, multiple sclerosis, phenytoin toxicity; rarely: hereditary ataxias.
- **Lower motor neurone dysarthria.** *Causes*: lesions of X (palatal), XII (tongue) or VII (facial): see relevant chapters.

 TIP   Some patients can have more than one type of dysarthria. For example, a patient with multiple sclerosis can have a combination of a cerebellar and spastic dysarthria.

3

MENTAL STATE AND HIGHER FUNCTION

1. MENTAL STATE

BACKGROUND

In this section, examination of higher function has been separated from examination of mental state. This is because higher function can be examined using relatively simple tests, while mental state is examined using observation of the patient and attention to points within the history.

The mental state relates to the mood and thoughts of a patient. Abnormalities may reflect:

- **neurological disease**, such as frontal lobe disease or dementia
- **psychiatric illness** which may be causing neurological symptoms (e.g. anxiety leading to panic attacks)
- **psychiatric illness** secondary to neurological disease (e.g. depression following stroke).

Mental state examination attempts to distinguish:

- focal neurological deficit
- diffuse neurological deficit
- primary psychiatric illness such as depression or anxiety presenting with somatic symptoms
- psychiatric illness secondary to, or associated with, neurological disease.

The extent of mental-state testing will depend on the patient and his problem. In many patients, only a simple assessment will be needed. However, it pays to consider whether further evaluation is needed in all patients.

Methods of formal psychiatric assessment will not be dealt with here.

WHAT TO DO AND WHAT YOU FIND

Appearance and behaviour

Watch the patient while you take the history. Here are some questions you can ask yourself in assessing appearance and behaviour.

Are there signs of self-neglect?

- Dirty or unkempt: consider depression, dementia, alcoholism or drug abuse.

Does the patient appear depressed?

- Furrowed brow, immobile, downcast facies, slow monotonous speech (cf. parkinsonism, Chapter 24).

Does the patient appear anxious?

- Fidgety, restless, with poor concentration.

Does the patient behave appropriately?

- Overfamiliar and disinhibited or aggressive: consider *frontalism*.
- Unresponsive, with little emotional response: *flat affect*.

Does the patient's mood change rapidly?

- Crying or laughing easily: *emotional lability.*

Does the patient show appropriate concern about his symptoms and disability?

- Lack of concern in the face of significant disability ('belle indifférence'): consider whether this reflects (i) *loss of insight and frontalism* or (ii) *conversion disorder*.

Mood

Ask the patient about his mood.

- How are your spirits at the moment?
- How would you describe your mood?

If you consider that the patient may be depressed, ask:

- During the past month have you often been bothered by:

    a) feeling down, depressed or hopeless?
    b) little interest or pleasure in doing things?

- Is this something with which you would like help?

A positive response to either (a) or (b) along with a request for help is a sensitive and specific screening test for depression.

Patients with schizophrenia often have an apparent lack of mood—*blunted affect*—or inappropriate mood, smiling when you expect them to be sad—*incongruous affect*.

In mania, patients are euphoric.

Vegetative symptoms

Ask the patient about vegetative symptoms:

- weight loss or gain
- sleep disturbance (waking early or difficulty getting to sleep)
- appetite
- constipation
- libido.

Look for symptoms of anxiety:

- palpitations
- sweating
- hyperventilation (tingling in fingers, in toes and around the mouth, dry mouth, dizziness and often a feeling of breathlessness).

Delusions

A delusion is a firmly held belief, not altered by rational argument, and not a conventional belief within the culture and society of the patient.

Delusional ideas may be revealed in the history but cannot be elicited by direct questioning. They can be classified according to their form (e.g. persecutory, grandiose, hypochondriacal) as well as by describing their content.

Delusions are seen in acute confusional states and psychotic illnesses.

Hallucinations and illusions

When a patient complains that he has seen, heard, felt or smelt something, you must decide whether it is an illusion or a hallucination.

An illusion is a misinterpretation of external stimuli and it is particularly common in patients with altered consciousness. For example, a confused patient says he can see a giant fist shaking outside the window, which is in fact a tree blowing in the wind outside.

A hallucination is a perception experienced without external stimuli that is indistinguishable from the perception of a real external stimulus.

Hallucinations may be *elementary*—flashes of light, bangs, whistles—or complex—seeing people, faces, hearing voices or music. Elementary hallucinations are usually organic.

Hallucinations can be described according to the type of sensation:

- *smell*: olfactory
- *taste*: gustatory—usually organic
- *sight*: visual
- *touch*: somatic—usually psychiatric
- *hearing*: auditory.

Before continuing, describe your findings, for example: 'An elderly unkempt man, who responds slowly but appropriately to questions and appears depressed'.

WHAT IT MEANS

In psychiatric diagnoses there is a hierarchy, and the psychiatric diagnosis is taken from the highest level involved. For example, a patient with both anxiety (low-level symptom) and psychotic symptoms (higher-level symptom) would be considered to have a psychosis (Table 3.1).

Organic psychoses

An organic psychosis is a neurological deficit producing an altered mental state, suggested by altered consciousness, fluctuating level of consciousness, disturbed memory, visual, olfactory, somatic and gustatory hallucinations, and sphincter disturbance.

Proceed to test higher function for localising signs.

There are three major syndromes:

- **Delirium or acute confusional state.** *Common causes*: drug-induced (especially sedative drugs, including antidepressants and antipsychotics), metabolic disturbances (especially hypoglycaemia), alcohol withdrawal, seizure-related (post-ictal or temporal lobe seizures).
- **Dysmnesic syndromes**: prominent loss of short-term memory, e.g. Korsakoff's psychosis (thiamine deficiency).
- **Dementia.** *Common causes*: given below (after higher function testing).

Functional psychoses

- **Schizophrenia**: clear consciousness, flat or incongruous affect, concrete thinking (see below), prominent delusions, formed auditory hallucinations, usually voices, which may speak to or

Table 3.1
Psychiatric diagnosis hierarchy

Highest	
Organic psychoses	
Functional psychoses	Schizophrenia
	Psychotic depression
	Bipolar (manic) depression
Neuroses	Depression
	Anxiety states
	Conversion disorders
	Phobias
	Obsessional neurosis
Personality disorders	
Lowest	

about the patient. May feel he is being controlled. May adopt strange postures and stay in them (catatonia).

- **Psychotic depression**: clear consciousness, depressed affect, no longer self-caring, slow, reports delusions (usually self-deprecating) or hallucinations. Usually vegetative symptoms: early waking, weight loss, reduced appetite, loss of libido, constipation. N.B. Considerable overlap with neurotic depression.
- **Bipolar depression**: episodes of depression as above, but also episodes of mania—elevated mood, grandiose delusions, pressure of speech and thought.

Neuroses

- **Depression**: low mood, loss of energy—following an identifiable event (e.g. bereavement). Vegetative symptoms less prominent.
- **Anxiety state**: debilitating anxiety without reasonable cause, prone to panic attacks, may hyperventilate.
- **Conversion disorder**: unconscious production or increase of a disability, associated with an inappropriate reaction to disability. There may be a secondary gain. Disability often does not conform to anatomical patterns of neurological loss.
- **Phobias**: irrational fear of something—ranging from open spaces to spiders.
- **Obsessional states**: a thought repeatedly intrudes into the patient's consciousness, often forcing him to actions (compulsions)—for example, the thought that the patient is contaminated forces him to wash his hands repeatedly. Patients may develop rituals.

Personality disorder

This is a lifelong extreme form of the normal range of personalities. For example:

- lacking ability to form relationships, abnormally aggressive and irresponsible = *psychopathic personality*
- histrionic, deceptive, immature = *borderline personality disorder.*

2. HIGHER FUNCTION

BACKGROUND

Higher function is a term used to encompass language (see Chapter 2), thought, memory, understanding, perception and intellect.

There are many sophisticated tests of higher function. These can be applied to test intelligence as well as in disease. However, much can be learned from simple bedside testing.

The purpose of testing is to:

- document the level of function in a reproducible way
- distinguish focal and diffuse deficits
- assess functional level within the community.

Higher function can be divided into the following elements:

- attention
- memory (immediate, short-term and long-term)
- calculation
- abstract thought
- spatial perception
- visual and body perception.

All testing relies on intact speech. This should be tested first. The tests cannot be interpreted if the patient has poor attention, as clearly this will interfere with all other aspects of testing. Results need to be interpreted in the light of premorbid intelligence. For example, the significance of an error in calculation clearly differs when found in a labourer and in a professor of mathematics.

WHEN TO TEST HIGHER FUNCTION

When should you test higher function formally? Obviously if the patient complains of loss of memory or of any alteration in higher function, you should proceed. In other patients the clues that should lead you to test come from the history. Patients are often remarkably adept at covering their loss of memory; vague answers to specific questions, and inconsistencies given without apparent concern, may suggest the need for testing. If in doubt, test. History from the relatives and friends is essential.

When you test higher function, the tests should be applied as:

1. an investigative tool directed towards the problem
2. screening tests to look for evidence of involvement of other higher functions.

For example, if a patient complains of poor memory, the examiner should test attention, short-term memory and longer-term memory, and then screen for involvement of calculation, abstract thought and spatial orientation.

 TIP   If the patient keeps turning to his partner looking for answers when you ask questions (the head-turning sign), this can indicate memory problems.

WHAT TO DO

Introduction

Before starting, explain that you are going to ask a number of questions. Apologise for the fact that some of these questions may seem very simple.

Test attention, orientation, memory and calculation whenever you test higher function. The other tests should be applied more selectively; indications will be outlined.

1. Attention and orientation

Orientation

Test orientation in time, place and person:

- *Time*: What day is it? What is the date? What is the month, the year? What is the season? What is the time of day?
- *Place*: What is the name of the place we are in? What is the name of the ward/hospital? What is the name of the town/city?
- *Person*: What is your name? What is your job? Where do you live?

Make a note of errors made.

Attention
Digit span
Tell the patient that you want him to repeat some numbers that you give him. Start with three- or four-digit numbers and increase until the patient makes several mistakes at one number of digits. Then explain that you want him to repeat the numbers backwards—for example, 'When I say one, two, three you say three, two, one.'

Note the number of digits the patient is able to recall forwards and backwards.

- *Normal*: seven forwards, five backwards.

 TIP   Use parts of telephone numbers you know (not 999 or your own!).

---

2. Memory

a. Immediate recall and attention
Name and address test
Tell the patient that you want him to remember a name and address. Use the type of address that the patient would be familiar with, e.g. 'John Brown, 5 Rose Cottages, Ruislip' or 'Jim Green, 20 Woodland Road, Chicago'. Ask him immediately to repeat it back to you.

Note how many errors are made in repeating it and how many times you have to repeat it before it is repeated correctly.

- *Normal*: immediate registration.

 TIP Develop a name and address that you use regularly so you do not make mistakes yourself.

Alternative test: Babcock sentence
Ask the patient to repeat this sentence: 'One thing a nation must have to be rich and great is a large, secure supply of wood.'

- *Normal*: correct in three attempts.

b. Short-term memory or episodic memory
About 5 minutes after asking the patient to remember the name and address, ask him to repeat it.
Note how many mistakes are made.

 TIP The 5 minutes can be spent testing calculation and abstract thought.

c. Long-term memory or semantic memory
Test factual knowledge you would expect the patient to have. This varies greatly from patient to patient and you need to tailor your questions accordingly. For example, a retired soldier should know the Commander-in-Chief in the Second World War, a football fan the year England won the World Cup, a neurologist the names of the cranial nerves. The following may be used as examples of general knowledge: dates of the Second World War, an American president who was shot dead.

3. Calculation

Serial sevens
Ask the patient if he is good with numbers, explaining that you are going to ask him to do some simple calculations. Ask him to take seven from a hundred, then seven from what remains.
Note mistakes and the time taken to perform calculation. N.B. These tests require good concentration, and poor performance may reflect impaired attention.

Alternative test: doubling threes
This should be used especially if serial sevens prove too difficult and if the patient professes difficulty with calculations. What is two times three? Twice that? And keep on doubling.
Note how high the patient is able to go and how long it takes.

Further tests
Ask the patient to perform increasingly difficult mental arithmetic: $2+3; 7+12; 21-9; 4\times7; 36\div9$ etc.

   N.B. Adjust to premorbid expectations.

4. Abstract thought

This tests for frontal lobe function: useful with frontal lobe lesions, dementia and psychiatric illness.

Tell the patient that you would like him to explain some proverbs to you.

   – **Ask him to explain well-known proverbs.** For example: 'A rolling stone gathers no moss', 'People in glass houses shouldn't throw stones', 'A stitch in time saves nine.'
   – **Does he give the correct interpretation?**

What you find
- Correct interpretation: *normal.*
- Physical interpretation: for example, the stone just rolls down so moss doesn't stick, or throwing stones will break the glass. This indicates *concrete thinking.*

Ask him to explain the difference between pairs of objects: e.g. a skirt and a pair of trousers, a table and a chair.
Ask the patient to estimate: the length of a jumbo jet (70 m or 230 feet); the weight of an elephant (5 tonnes); the height of the Eiffel Tower (986 feet or 300 m); the number of camels in The Netherlands (some in zoos).

What you find
- Reasonable estimates: *normal.*
- Unreasonable estimates: indicates *abnormal abstract thinking.*

5. Spatial perception

This tests for parietal and occipital lobe function.

Clock face
Ask the patient to draw a clock face and to fill in the numbers. Ask him then to draw the hands on at a given time: for example, ten to four.

Five-pointed star
Ask the patient to copy a five-pointed star (Fig. 3.1).

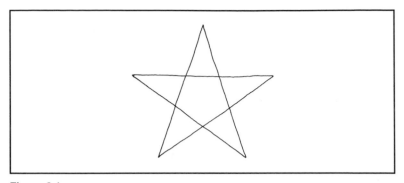

Figure 3.1
Five-pointed star

What you find
- Accurate clock and star: *normal*.
- Half clock missing: *visual inattention*.
- Unable to draw clock or reproduce star: *constructional apraxia*.

 TIP This is difficult to assess in the presence of weakness.

6. Visual and body perception

Tests for parietal and occipital lesions.

Abnormalities of perception of sensation despite normal sensory pathways are called *agnosias*. Agnosias can occur in all modalities of sensation but in clinical practice they usually affect vision, touch and body perception.

The sensory pathway needs to have been examined and found to be intact before a patient is considered to have an agnosia. However, agnosia is usually regarded as part of higher function and is therefore considered here.

Facial recognition: 'famous faces'
Take a bedside newspaper or magazine and ask the patient to identify the faces of famous people. Choose people the patient will be expected to know: the US President, the Queen, the Prime Minister, film stars and so on.
Note mistakes made.

- Recognises faces: *normal*.
- Does not recognise faces: *prosopagnosia*.

Body perception
- Patient ignores one side (usually the left) and is unable to find his hand if asked (*hemi-neglect*).
- Patient does not recognise his left hand if shown it (*asomatagnosia*).

- Patient is unaware of weakness of the affected (usually left) side (*anosagnosia*)—and will often move the right side when asked to move the left.

Ask the patient to show you his index finger, ring finger and so on.

- Failure: finger agnosia.

Ask the patient to touch his right ear with his left index finger. Cross your hands and ask which is your right hand.

- Failure: left/right agnosia.

Sensory agnosia

Ask the patient to close his eyes. Place an object—e.g. coin, key, paperclip—in his hand and ask him what it is.

- Failure: astereognosis.

Ask the patient to close his eyes. Write a number or letter on his hand and ask him what it is.

- Failure: agraphaesthesia.

 TIP   Test on the unaffected side first, to ensure the patient understands the test.

---

7. Apraxia

Apraxia is a term used to describe an inability to perform a task when there is no weakness, incoordination or movement disorder to prevent it. It will be described here, though clearly examination of the motor system is required before it can be assessed.

Tests for parietal lobe and premotor cortex of the frontal lobe function.

Ask the patient to perform an imaginary task: 'Show me how you would comb your hair, drink a cup of tea, strike a match and blow it out.' **Observe the patient.** If there is a difficulty, give the patient an appropriate object and see if he is able to perform the task with the appropriate prompt. If there is further difficulty, demonstrate and ask him to copy what you are doing.

- The patient is able to perform the act appropriately: *normal.*
- The patient is unable to initiate the action though understanding the command: *ideational apraxia.*
- The patient performs the task but makes errors: for example, uses his hand as a cup rather than holding an imaginary cup: *ideomotor apraxia.*

If inability is related to a specific task—for example, dressing—this should be referred to as a dressing apraxia. This is often tested in hospital by asking the patient to put on a dressing gown with one sleeve pulled inside out. The patient should normally be able to overcome this easily.

Three-hand test

Ask the patient to copy your hand movements and demonstrate: (1) make a fist and tap it on the table with your thumb upwards; (2) then straighten out your fingers and tap on the table with your thumb upwards; (3) then place your palm flat on the table. If the patient is unable to perform this after one demonstration, repeat the demonstration.

- If the patient is unable to perform this in the presence of normal motor function: *limb apraxia.*

WHAT YOU FIND

Three patterns can be recognised:

- **Patients with poor attention.** Tests are useful to document level of function, but are of limited use in distinguishing focal from diffuse disease. Further assessment is discussed in Chapter 27.
- **Patients with deficits in many or all major areas of testing.** Indicates a diffuse or multifocal process.
  - If of slow onset: dementia or chronic brain syndrome.
  - If of more rapid onset: confusional state or acute brain syndrome.

COMMON MISTAKES

Dementia needs to be distinguished from:

- **low intelligence**: usually indicated from a history of intellectual attainment
- **depression**: may be difficult, especially in the elderly. Often suggested by the patient's demeanour
- **aphasia**: usually found on critical testing.

- **Patients with deficits in one or only a few areas of testing.** Indicates a focal process. Identify the area affected and seek associated physical signs (Table 3.2).

Patterns of focal loss

- **Impaired attention and orientation**: occurs with diffuse disturbance of cerebral function. *If acute,* often associated with disturbance of consciousness; assess as Chapter 27. *If chronic,* limits ability for further testing; this is suggestive of dementia. N.B. Also occurs with anxiety and depression.
- **Memory**: loss of short-term memory in alert patient—usually bilateral, limbic system (hippocampus, mamillary bodies) disturbance—seen in diffuse encephalopathies; bilateral temporal lesions; prominent in Korsakoff's psychosis (thiamine deficiency). Loss of long-term memory with preserved short-term memory: functional memory loss.

Table 3.2
Patterns of focal loss

Lobe	Alteration in higher function	Associations
Frontal	Apathy, disinhibition	Contralateral hemiplegia, Broca's aphasia (dominant hemisphere), primitive reflexes
Temporal	Memory	Wernicke's aphasia (dominant hemisphere), upper quadrantanopia
Parietal	Calculation, perceptual and spatial orientation (non-dominant hemisphere)	Apraxia (dominant hemisphere), homonymous hemianopia, hemisensory disturbance, neglect
Occipital	Perceptual and spatial orientation	Hemianopia

- **Calculation**: impaired calculation usually indicates diffuse encephalopathy. If associated with finger agnosia (inability to name fingers), left–right agnosia (inability to distinguish left from right) and dysgraphia=Gerstmann syndrome—indicates a dominant parietal lobe syndrome. Perverse but consistent calculation errors may suggest psychiatric disease.
- **Abstract thought**: if interpretations of proverbs are concrete— suggests diffuse encephalopathy. If interpretation includes delusional ideas—suggests psychiatric illness, with particular frontal lobe involvement. Poor estimates suggest frontal or diffuse encephalopathy or psychiatric illness.
- **Loss of spatial appreciation**: (copying drawings, astereognosis)— parietal lobe lesions.
- **Visual and body perception**:
  - Prosopagnosia: bilateral temporoparietal lesions.
  - Neglect
  - Sensory agnosia   } parietal lobe lesions.
  - Astereognosis
  - Agraphaesthesia
- **Apraxia:**
  - Ideomotor apraxia: lesion of either the dominant parietal lobe or premotor cortex, or a diffuse brain lesion.
  - Ideational apraxia: suggests bilateral parietal disease.

WHAT IT MEANS

Diffuse or multifocal abnormalities

Common
- Alzheimer's disease.
- Vascular disease (multi-infarct).

Rare
Degenerative conditions
- Pick's disease.
- Frontotemporal dementia.
- Diffuse Lewy body disease.
- Huntington's disease.

Nutritional
- Thiamine deficiency (Korsakoff's psychosis).
- Vitamin B_{12} deficiency.

Infective
- Quaternary syphilis.
- Creutzfeldt–Jakob disease.
- HIV encephalopathy.

Structural
- Normal pressure hydrocephalus.
- Demyelination.
- Multiple sclerosis.

Focal deficits

May indicate early stage of a multifocal disease.

Vascular
- Thrombosis, emboli or haemorrhage.

Neoplastic
- Primary or secondary tumours.

Infective
- Abscess.

Demyelinating
- Multiple sclerosis.

4

GAIT

BACKGROUND

Always examine the patient's gait. It is a coordinated action requiring integration of sensory and motor functions. The gait may be the only abnormality on examination, or it may lead you to seek appropriate clinical associations on the rest of the examination. The most commonly seen are: hemiplegic, parkinsonian, marche à petits pas, ataxic and unsteady gaits.

Romberg's test is conveniently performed after examining the gait. This is a simple test primarily of joint position sense.

WHAT TO DO AND WHAT YOU FIND

Ask the patient to walk.
Ensure you are able to see the arms and legs adequately.
Is the gait symmetrical?

- Yes: see Figures 4.1 and 4.2.
- No: see below.

(Gaits can usually be divided into symmetrical and asymmetrical even though the symmetry is not perfect.)

If symmetrical
Look at the size of paces:

- Small or normal?

If small paces:
Look at the posture and arm-swing:

- Stooped with reduced arm-swing: *parkinsonian* (may be difficult to start and stop: *festinant*—may be worse on one side; tremor may be seen to increase on walking). Reduced arm-swing, usually unilateral, is one of the earliest signs of parkinsonism.
- Upright with marked arm-swing: *marche à petits pas.*

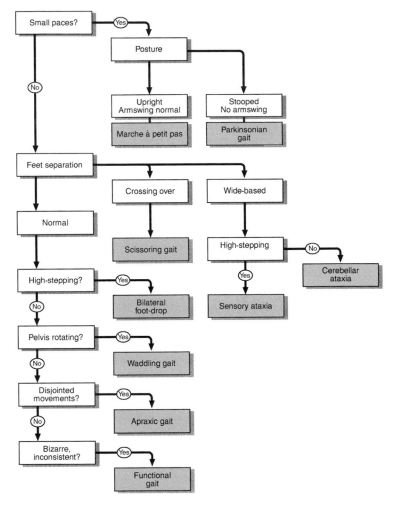

Figure 4.1
Flow chart: gait

If normal paces:
Look at the lateral distance between the feet:

- Normal.
- Widely separated: *broad-based.*
- Legs uncoordinated: *cerebellar.*
- Crossing over, toes dragged: *scissoring.*

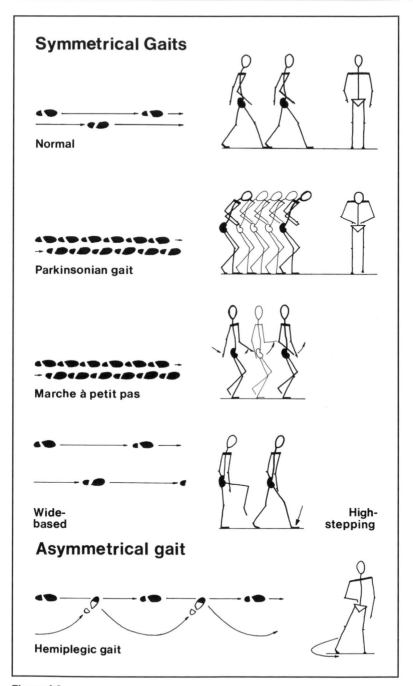

Symmetrical Gaits

Normal

Parkinsonian gait

Marche à petit pas

Wide-based

High-stepping

Asymmetrical gait

Hemiplegic gait

Figure 4.2
Gaits

Look at the knees:

- Normal.
- Knees lifted high: *high-stepping.*

Look at the pelvis and shoulders:

- Normal.
- Marked rotation of pelvis and shoulder: *waddling.*

Look at the whole movement:

- Normal.
- Disjointed as if the patient has forgotten how to walk and he frequently appears rooted to the spot: *apraxic.*
- Bizarre, elaborate and inconsistent: *functional.*

If asymmetrical

Is the patient in pain?

- Yes: painful or antalgic gait.

Look for a bony deformity:

- Orthopaedic gait.

Does one leg swing out to the side?

- Yes: hemiplegic gait.

Look at the knee heights:

- Normal.
- One knee lifts higher: *foot drop.*

FURTHER TESTS

Ask the patient to walk as if on a tight-rope (*demonstrate*).

- If patient falls consistently: *unsteady.*
- May fall predominantly to one side.
- Elderly patients are often slightly unsteady.

Ask the patient to walk on his heels (*demonstrate*).

- If unable to: *foot drop.*

Ask the patient to walk on his toes (*demonstrate*).

- If unable to: weakness of gastrocnemius.

WHAT IT MEANS

- **Parkinsonian**: indicates basal ganglion dysfunction. *Common causes*: Parkinson's disease, major tranquillisers.

- **Marche à petits pas**: indicates bilateral diffuse cortical dysfunction. *Common cause*: diffuse cerebrovascular disease 'lacunar state'.
- **Scissoring**: indicates spastic paraparesis. *Common causes*: cerebral palsy, multiple sclerosis, cord compression.
- **Sensory ataxia**: indicates loss of joint position sense (Romberg's positive). *Common causes*: peripheral neuropathy, posterior column loss (see below).
- **Cerebellar ataxia**: veers towards side of lesion. *Common causes*: drugs (e.g. phenytoin), alcohol, multiple sclerosis, cerebrovascular disease.
- **Waddling gait**: indicates weak or ineffective proximal muscles. *Common causes*: proximal myopathies, bilateral congenital dislocation of the hip.
- **Apraxic gait**: indicates that cortical integration of the movement is abnormal, usually with frontal lobe pathology. *Common causes*: normal pressure hydrocephalus, cerebrovascular disease.
- **Hemiplegic**: unilateral upper motor neurone lesion. *Common causes*: stroke, multiple sclerosis.
- **Foot drop**: *Common causes*: unilateral—common peroneal palsy, pyramidal lesion, L5 radiculopathy; bilateral—peripheral neuropathy.
- **Functional gait**: variable, may be inconsistent with rest of examination, worse when watched. May be mistaken for the gait in chorea (especially Huntington's disease), which is shuffling, twitching and spasmodic and has associated findings on examination (see Chapter 24).

Non-neurological gaits

- **Painful gait**: *Common causes*: arthritis, trauma—usually obvious.
- **Orthopaedic gait**: *Common causes*: shortened limb, previous hip surgery, trauma.

Romberg's test

What to do
Ask the patient to stand with his feet together.

- Allow him to stand like this for a few seconds.

Tell the patient you are ready to catch him if he falls (make sure you are).

- If he falls with his eyes open, you cannot proceed with the test.

If not:

Ask the patient to close his eyes.

What you find and what it means
- Stands with eyes open; stands with eyes closed = Romberg's test is negative: *normal*.

- Stands with eyes open; falls with eyes closed=Romberg's test is positive: *loss of joint position sense*. This can occur with:
  - Posterior column lesion in the spinal cord: *Common causes*: cord compression (e.g. cervical spondylosis, tumour). *Rarer causes*: tabes dorsalis, vitamin B_{12} deficiency, degenerative spinal cord disease.
  - Peripheral neuropathy: *Common causes*: see Chapter 20.
- **Unable to stand with eyes open and feet together**=severe unsteadiness. *Common causes*: cerebellar syndromes and both central and peripheral vestibular syndromes.
- **Stands with eyes open; rocks backwards and forwards with eyes closed**: suggests a cerebellar syndrome.

COMMON MISTAKES

- Romberg's test *cannot* be performed if the patient cannot stand unaided.
- Romberg's test is *not* positive in cerebellar disease.

CRANIAL NERVES:

5

GENERAL

BACKGROUND

Abnormalities found when examining the 'cranial nerves' may arise from lesions at different levels (Fig. 5.1) including:

a. the central nervous system pathways to and from the cortex, diencephalon (thalamus and associated structures), cerebellum or other parts of the brainstem
b. lesions in the nucleus
c. lesions to the nerve itself
d. generalised problems of nerve, neuromuscular junction or muscle.

When examining the cranial nerves, you need to establish whether there is an abnormality in cranial nerve function, the nature and extent of the abnormality and any associations.

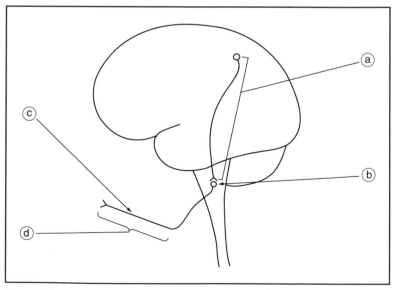

Figure 5.1
Location of cranial nerve abnormalities (see text for key)

COMMON MISTAKES

Sometimes, when summarising neurological examination, people divide it into 'cranial nerves' and examination of the 'peripheral nervous system'. This distinction misleads. By thinking of the examination in this way, you can forget that you are examining not just the cranial or peripheral nerves but also their central nervous system connections. To prevent ensnaring yourself in this trap, it is useful to think of examination of the 'head and neck' rather than the 'cranial nerves', and the 'limbs' rather than the 'peripheral nervous system'. Tradition is so strong that this book continues to describe examination under the heading 'cranial nerves', but you know better…

More than one cranial nerve may be abnormal:

- if there is a lesion where several cranial nerves run together either in the brainstem or within the skull (e.g. cerebellopontine angle or cavernous sinus)
- when affected by a generalised disorder (e.g. myasthenia gravis)
- following multiple lesions (e.g. multiple sclerosis, cerebrovascular disease, basal meningitis).

Abnormalities of cranial nerves are very useful in localising a lesion within the central nervous system.

Examination of the eye and its fields allows the examination of a tract running from the eye to the occipital lobe that also crosses the midline.

The nuclei of the cranial nerves within the brainstem act as markers for the level of the lesion (Fig. 5.2). Particularly useful are the nuclei of the III, IV, VI, VII and XII nerves. When the tongue and face are affected on the same side as a hemiplegia, the lesion must be above the XII and VII nucleus respectively. If a cranial nerve is affected on the opposite side to a hemiparesis, then the causative lesion must be at the level of the nucleus of that nerve. This is illustrated in Figure 5.3.

Multiple cranial nerve abnormalities are also recognised in a number of syndromes:

- Unilateral V, VII and VIII: cerebellopontine angle lesion.
- Unilateral III, IV, V_1 and VI: cavernous sinus lesion.
- Combined unilateral IX, X and XI: jugular foramen syndrome.
  - Combined bilateral X, XI and XII:
  - if *lower motor neurone*=bulbar palsy
  - if *upper motor neurone*=pseudobulbar palsy.
- Prominent involvement of eye muscles and facial weakness, particularly when variable, suggests a myasthenic syndrome.

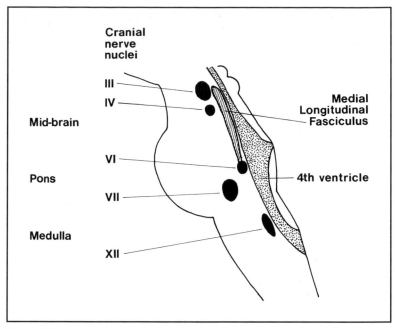

Figure 5.2
Level of cranial nerve nuclei in the brainstem, indicated by roman numerals

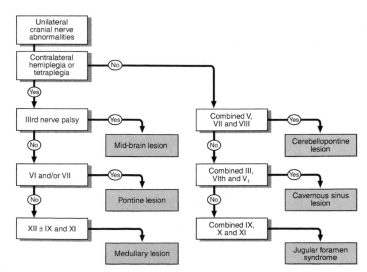

Figure 5.3
Flow chart: multiple cranial nerve abnormalities

- Multiple cranial nerve palsies can reflect basal meningitis—either malignant meningitis, chronic infective or inflammatory meningitis.

The most common cause of intrinsic brainstem lesions in younger patients is multiple sclerosis, and in older patients it is vascular disease. Rarer causes include gliomas, lymphomas and brainstem encephalitis.

 TIP If you think a patient has multiple cranial nerve palsies, ask yourself whether they might have myasthenia… and look for fatigable weakness.

CRANIAL NERVE I: 6

OLFACTORY NERVE

This is rarely tested in clinical practice.

Examination is usually performed to investigate a specific complaint rather than as a screening test. Most recognisable smells require olfaction. Some agents such as ammonia can be recognised by the nasal epithelium and do not require an intact olfactory pathway.

WHAT TO DO

- **Very simple**: Ask the patient if they have noticed a change in their sense of smell (this is really history rather than examination).
- **Simple**: Take a bedside object—a piece of fruit, an orange, a juice bottle—and ask the patient if it smells normal.
- **Formal**: A selection of substances with identifiable smells in similar bottles is used. Agents often used include peppermint, camphor and rosewater. The subject is asked to identify these smells. An agent such as ammonia is usually included. Each nostril is tested separately.

WHAT YOU FIND

- The patient is able to identify smells appropriately: *normal.*
- The patient is unable to recognise scents offered but recognises ammonia: *anosmia.* This finding is limited to one nostril: *unilateral anosmia.*
- The patient recognises no smells, including ammonia: consider that the loss may not be entirely organic.

WHAT IT MEANS

- **Anosmia in both nostrils**: loss of sense of smell. *Common causes*: blocked nasal passages (e.g. common cold), trauma; a relative loss occurs with ageing and Parkinson's disease.
- **Unilateral anosmia**: blocked nostril, unilateral frontal lesion (meningioma or glioma—extremely rare).

CRANIAL NERVES: 7

THE EYE 1 – Pupils, Acuity, Fields

BACKGROUND

Examination of the eye can provide very many important diagnostic clues for both general medical and neurological diseases.

Examination can be divided into:

1. general
2. pupils
3. acuity
4. fields
5. fundi (next chapter).

2. Pupils

The pupillary light reaction

- *Afferent*: optic nerve.
- *Efferent*: parasympathetic component of the third nerve on both sides.

Accommodation reaction

- *Afferent*: arises in the frontal lobes.
- *Efferent*: as for light reaction.

3. Acuity

Abnormalities may arise from:

- **Ocular problems**, such as dense cataracts (lens opacities). These are not correctable with glasses but are readily identifiable on ophthalmoscopy.
- **Optical problems**: abnormalities of the focal length of the focusing system in the eye, commonly called long- or short-sightedness.

These can be corrected by glasses or by asking the patient to look through a pinhole.

- **Retinal or retro-orbital abnormality of vision** which cannot be corrected using lenses. Retinal causes are often visible on ophthalmoscopy.

It is essential to test acuity with the patient's correct glasses.

4. Fields

The organisation of the visual pathways means different patterns of visual field abnormality arise from lesions at different sites. The normal visual pathways are given in Figure 7.1.

The visual fields are divided vertically through the point of fixation into the temporal and nasal fields. Something on your right as you look ahead is in the temporal field of your right eye and the nasal field of your left eye.

The visual fields are described from the patient's point of view.

Field defects are said to be homonymous if the same part of the visual field is affected in both eyes. This can be congruous (the field defects in both eyes match exactly) or incongruous (the field defects do not match exactly).

Testing the fields is very useful in localisation of a lesion (Table 7.1).

The normal visual fields for different types of stimuli are very different. The normal field for moving objects or large objects is wider than for objects held still or small objects. The normal field for recognition of coloured objects is more limited than for monochrome. It is useful to test this on yourself. Look straight into the distance in front of you and put your hands out straight to your side. Wiggle your fingers and, keeping your arms straight, gradually bring your arms forward until you can see your moving fingers. Repeat this holding a small white object, and then with a red object until you can see that it is red. You will appreciate the different normal fields for these different stimuli.

Table 7.1
Testing the visual fields

Type of defect	Site of lesion
Monocular field defect	Anterior to optic chiasm
Bitemporal field defect	At the optic chiasm
Homonymous field defect	Behind the optic chiasm
Congruous homonymous field defect	Behind the lateral geniculate bodies

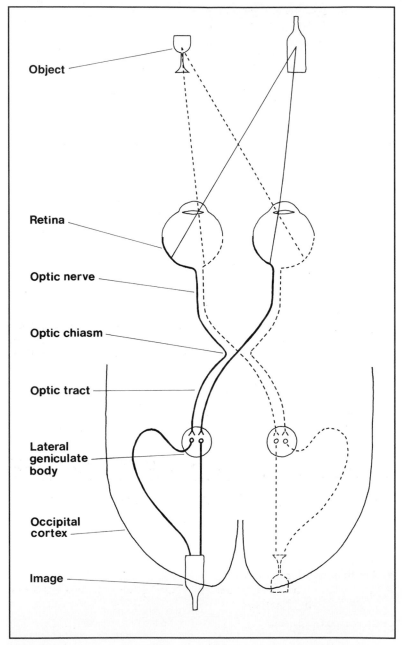

Figure 7.1
Visual pathways

1. GENERAL

WHAT TO DO

Look at the patient's eyes and note any difference between the two sides.
Look at the level of the eyelid; particularly note asymmetry.

- If an eyelid is lower than normal, this is referred to as *ptosis*; it can be *partial* or *complete* (if eye is closed).
- If an eyelid is higher than normal, usually above the level of the top of the iris, this is described as *lid retraction*.

Look at the position of the eye.

- Is there protrusion (*exophthalmos*) or does the eye appear sunken (*enophthalmos*)? If you are considering exophthalmos, it is confirmed if the front of the orbital globe can be seen when looking from above.

  Beware the false eye—usually obvious on closer inspection.

WHAT IT MEANS

- **Ptosis.** *Common causes*: congenital, Horner's syndrome (ptosis always partial), third nerve palsy (ptosis often complete) (see below); in older patients, the levator muscles can become weak or detached from the lid, producing age-related ptosis. *Rarer causes*: myasthenia gravis (ptosis often variable), myopathy.
- **Exophthalmos.** *Common causes*: most frequently, dysthyroid eye disease—associated with lid retraction. *Rarely*: retro-orbital mass.
- **Enophthalmos:** a feature of Horner's syndrome (see below).

2. PUPILS

WHAT TO DO IN A CONSCIOUS PATIENT

(For pupillary changes in an unconscious patient, see Chapter 27.)
Look at the pupils.

- Are they equal in size?
- Are they regular in outline?
- Are there any holes in the iris or foreign bodies (e.g. lens implants) in the anterior chamber?

Shine a bright light in one eye.

- Look at the reaction of that eye—the direct reflex—and then repeat and look at the reaction in the other eye—the consensual reflex.

- Ensure that the patient is **looking into the distance** and not at the light.
- Repeat for the other eye.

Place your finger 10 cm in front of the patient's nose. Ask the patient to **look into the distance and then at your finger.**
Look at the pupils for their reaction to *accommodation.*

WHAT YOU FIND

See Figure 7.2.

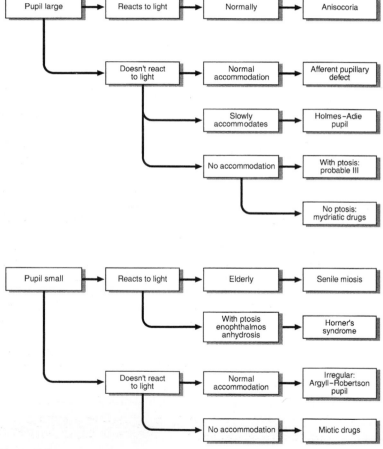

Figure 7.2
Flow chart: pupillary abnormalities

FURTHER TESTING
Swinging light test
What to do
Shine a bright light into one eye and then the other at about 1-second intervals. Swing the light repeatedly between the two. Observe the pupillary response as the light is shone into the eye.

What you find and what it means
- The pupil constricts as the light is shone into it repeatedly: normal.
- The pupil on one side constricts when the light is shone into it and the pupil on the other side dilates when the light is then shone into it: the side that dilates has a relative afferent pupillary defect (often abbreviated to RAPD). This is also sometimes called the Marcus Gunn pupil. N.B. This lesion is always unilateral.

WHAT IT MEANS
- **Anisocoria**: pupils unequal but normally reacting—normal variant.
- **Senile miosis**: normal age-related change.
- **Holmes–Adie pupil**: degeneration of ciliary ganglion of unknown cause; may be associated with loss of tendon reflexes.
- **Afferent pupillary defect**: lesion anterior to the optic chiasm. *Common cause*: optic neuritis. *Rarer causes*: compression of the optic nerve, retinal degenerations.
- **Relative afferent pupillary defect**: partial lesion anterior to the optic chiasm. *Causes*: as for afferent pupillary defects.
- **Horner's syndrome** (miosis, partial ptosis, enophthalmos and loss of hemifacial sweating): lesion to sympathetic fibres. This may occur:
  - **Centrally**: in the hypothalamus, the medulla or the upper cervical cord (exits at T1). *Common cause*: stroke (N.B. lateral medullary syndrome), demyelination. *Rarely*: trauma or syringomyelia.
  - **Peripherally**: in the sympathetic chain, in the superior cervical ganglion or along the carotid artery. *Common causes*: Pancoast's tumour (apical bronchial carcinoma), trauma. *Rare cause*: carotid dissection. Sometimes no cause is found.
- **Argyll–Robertson pupil**: probably an upper midbrain lesion; now very rare. *Common causes*: syphilis, diabetes mellitus. *Rarely*: multiple sclerosis (MS).

3. ACUITY

WHAT TO DO AND WHAT YOU FIND
Can the patient see out of both eyes?
Ask the patient to **put on glasses** if used.

Cover one of the patient's eyes. Test each eye in turn.

Acuity can be tested in several ways.

(i) Using **Snellen's** chart
- Stand the patient 6m from a well-lit chart. Ask him to read down from the largest letters to the smallest.
- Record the results: distance in metres or feet from chart; distance in metres or feet at which letters should be seen.

For example: 6/6 when the letter is read at the correct distance or 6/60 when the largest letter (normally seen at 60m) is read at 6m, or 20/20 and 20/200 when these acuities are measured in feet.

(ii) Using a near vision chart (Fig. 7.3)
- Hold the chart 30cm from patient and ask him to read sections of print.
- Record the smallest print size read (e.g. N6).
- Ensure reading glasses are used if needed.

N.5.

Boat, house, horse, cat, cabbage, man, trousers, yellow.

N.6.

Eye, ear, earth, lion, lying, road, green, dog.

N.8.

Bird, wall, silver, tower, train, gorse.

N.10.

Snail, sail, blue, jacket, clam, jockey.

N.12.

Car, crow, grey, bracket, scarlet.

N.14.

White, bank, turbot, jewel.

N.18.

Play, grain, red, goat.

N.24.

Black, frog, tree.

Figure 7.3
Near vision chart

(iii) Using bedside material such as newspapers

Test as in (ii) and record the type size read (e.g. headlines only, all print).

If unable to read largest letters:
See if the patient can:

- **Count fingers.** Ask how many fingers you are holding up.
- **See hand movements.** Ask him to say when you move your hand in front of his eye.
- **Perceive light.** Ask him to say when you shine a light in his eye.

Ask the patient to **look through a pinhole** made in a card.

If acuity improves, the visual impairment is refractive in origin and not from other optical or neurological causes.

A new development

Ophthalmologists are increasingly using LogMAR (logarithm of the minimum angle of resolution) charts to measure acuity. There are a number of different LogMAR chart designs. They are read in the same way as a Snellen chart. However, the result is expressed as the logarithm of the minimum angle or resolution, which in turn is the inverse of the Snellen ratio. For example, for Snellen acuities:

6/6 or 20/20 = logMAR 0.0.
6/24 or 20/80 = logMAR +0.6
6/60 or 20/200 = logMAR +1.0.

WHAT IT MEANS

- Reduced acuity correctable by pinhole or glasses: refractive optical defect.
- Reduced acuity not correctable: classified according to site along the visual pathway—from the front of the eye back to the occipital cortex:

Anterior	Corneal lesion: ulceration, oedema
	Cataract
	Macular degeneration: especially age-related
	Retinal haemorrhage or infarct
	Optic neuropathy:
	– Inflammatory (MS)
	– Ischaemic
	– Compressive
	Retrochiasmal: macula-splitting field defect (see below)
	Bilateral occipital lesions: cortical blindness
Posterior	

4. FIELDS

WHAT TO DO

Assess major field defects

- Ask the patient to look with both eyes at your eyes.
- Put your hands out on both sides approximately 50 cm apart and approximately 30 cm above eye level. Extend your index finger (Fig. 7.4). Your fingers should now be in the patient's upper temporal fields on both sides.
- Ask the patient to indicate which index finger you move: right, left or both.
- Repeat with hands approximately 30 cm below eye level.

If one side is ignored when both fingers are moved together but is seen when moved by itself, then there is visual inattention.

Test each eye individually

What to test with?

Large objects are more easily seen than small objects; white objects are more easily seen than red. Thus, fields will vary according to the size and colour of the target used.

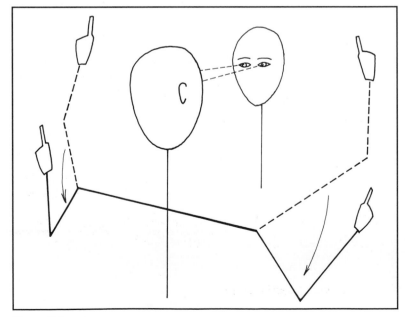

Figure 7.4
Screening for gross visual field defects

Central vision is colour (cones) and peripheral vision is mono-chrome (rods).

A combination of wiggling fingers (described above) and red pin provide the most sensitive and specific bedside test for field defects.

- Sit just under one arm's length away from the patient at the same level.
- Cover the patient's right eye and ask him to look at your right eye with his left eye. This is so you are certain of his point of fixation throughout the test.
- Tilt the patient's head to get the eyebrows and nose out of the way.

Using a red pin (recommended):
- Imagine there is a plane, like a vertical sheet of glass, halfway between you and the patient (Fig. 7.5A). You are going to compare your visual field on that plane with the patient's visual field on that plane. The field to red is about 30–40 degrees from the point of fixation.
- Hold the red pin within that plane beyond where you can see it as red. Move it within the plane towards the point of fixation. Ask the patient to tell you when he can **see it as red.**
- Bring the pin slowly from four directions: northeast, northwest, southeast and southwest (where north/south is the vertical). Compare the patient's visual field to your own.
- To find the blind spot, move the pin from the point of fixation halfway between you, laterally along the horizontal meridian until you find your own blind spot. Ask the patient to tell you when the pin disappears.

Alternative technique using a white pin:
- Imagine a sphere of radius 30 cm centred on the patient's eye.
- Bring a white pin in towards the line of fixation along an arc of a sphere centred on the patient's eye (Fig. 7.5B).
- Ensure the pin cannot be seen where you start (usually behind the plane of the eyes). Ask the patient to tell you when he first sees the pin.
- Initially bring the pin **slowly** from four directions, northeast, northwest, southeast and southwest (where north/south is the vertical).

Once you find a field defect
Define the edges.

Bring the pin from where it cannot be seen to where it can be seen.

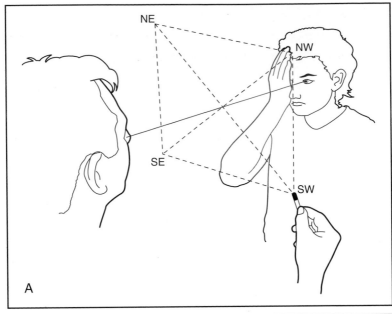

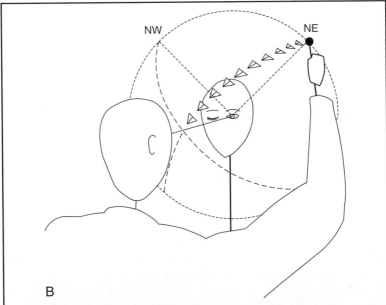

Figure 7.5
Testing peripheral visual fields. **A:** with a red pin; **B:** with a white pin

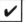 **TIP** The edges are often vertical or horizontal (Fig. 7.6).

When there is a homonymous hemianopia
The macula needs to be tested.

Bring the pin horizontally from the side with the defect towards the point of fixation.

• If the pin is seen before it gets to the midline, there is macular sparing.
• If the pin is only seen once it crosses the midline, there is no macular sparing.

Describe the field loss from the patient's point of view.

Central field defects—*scotomas*—and the *blind spot* (the field defect produced by the optic disc) are usually found using a red pin.

 TIP If a patient complains of a hole in his visual field, it is often easier to give him the pin and ask him to place it in the hole in his vision.

COMMON MISTAKES

• Upper temporal field defects: *eyebrows*
• Lower nasal field defects: *nose*
• Patient moves eyes ('cheats') *looking to one side: long-standing homonymous hemianopia* on that side

WHAT YOU FIND

See Figure 7.7.

(i) Defect limited to one eye

Constricted field
• **Tubular vision**: the size of the constricted field remains the same regardless of the distance of the test object from the eye.
• **Scotoma**: a hole in the visual field—described by its site (e.g. *central* or *centrocaecal*— defect connecting the fixation point to the blind spot) and shape (e.g. *round* or *ring-shaped*).
• **Altitudinal defect**: a lesion confined to either the upper or the lower half of the visual field but crossing the vertical meridian.

(ii) Defect affecting both eyes

• **Bitemporal hemianopias**: defect in the temporal fields of both eyes. Note carefully if the upper or lower quadrant is more marked.

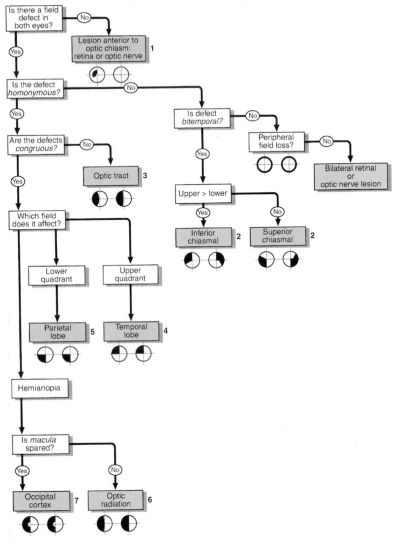

Figure 7.6
Flow chart: field defects

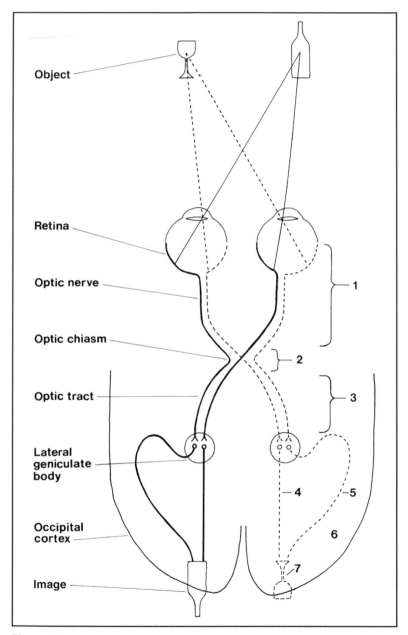

Figure 7.7
Visual pathways with sites of lesions marked. Numbers match those in Figure 7.6

- **Homonymous quadrantanopias**: defect in the same quadrant of vision of both eyes. Classified as *congruous* or *incongruous* (see above).
- **Homonymous hemianopias**: defect in the same hemifield in both eyes. Classified according to degree of functional preservation in the affected field (e.g. able to see moving targets), whether *congruous* or *incongruous,* and whether *macula-sparing* or not.
- **Others**, including bilateral defects as described in (i).

Describe your findings: for example, 'This man has normal pupillary response to light and accommodation. His visual acuities are 6/6 on the right and 6/12 on the left. He has a right homonymous hemianopia which is congruous and macula-sparing.'

WHAT IT MEANS

See Figures 7.6 and 7.7.

(i) *Defect limited to one eye*: indicates ocular, retinal or optic nerve pathology.

- **Constricted field**: chronic papilloedema, chronic glaucoma.
- **Tubular vision**: does not indicate organic disease—suggests conversion disorder.
- **Scotoma**: MS, toxic optic neuropathy, ischaemic optic neuropathy, retinal haemorrhage or infarct.
- **Enlarged blind spots**: papilloedema.
- **Altitudinal defects**: suggest vascular cause (retinal infarcts or ischaemic optic neuropathy).

(ii) *Defect affecting both eyes*: indicates a lesion at or behind the optic chiasm, or bilateral prechiasmal lesions.

- Bitemporal hemianopias
  - *Upper quadrant > lower*: inferior chiasmal compression, commonly a pituitary adenoma
  - *Lower quadrant > upper*: superior chiasmal compression, commonly a craniopharyngioma.

The common causes for the lesions referred to below are cerebral infarcts, haemorrhages, tumours or head injuries.

- **Homonymous** quadrantanopias
  - *Upper*: temporal lobe lesion
  - *Lower*: parietal lobe lesion.
- **Homonymous** hemianopias
  - *Incongruous*: lesion of the optic tract
  - *Congruous*: lesion behind the lateral geniculate body
  - *Macula-sparing*: lesion of the occipital cortex (or partial lesion of optic tract or radiation).

CRANIAL NERVES: **8**

THE EYE 2 – Fundi

BACKGROUND

The ophthalmoscope provides a light source and an optical system to allow examination of the fundus (Fig. 8.1).

Its moving parts are:

- on/off switch, usually with brightness control
- focus ring (occasionally two)
- sometimes a beam selector
- sometimes a dust cover.

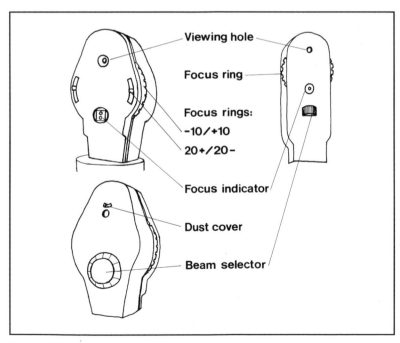

Figure 8.1
The parts of two commonly used ophthalmoscopes

The **focus ring** is used to correct (1) for your vision and (2) for the patient's vision.

1. If you are short- or near-sighted (*myopic*) and not using glasses or contact lenses, you will have to turn the focus dial anticlockwise to focus to look at a normal eye; turn it clockwise if you are long- or far-sighted (*hypermetropic*). Establish what correction you need before approaching the patient.
2. If the patient is myopic, turn the ring anticlockwise; if hypermetropic, clockwise.

 TIP An oblique view of the patient with his spectacles on tells you if he is long- or short-sighted and gives an idea of severity. If his face is smaller through his glasses, he is myopic; if his face is larger, he is hypermetropic. The degree indicates severity.

Beam selector choices are:

- standard for general use
- narrow beam for looking at the macula
- target (like a rifle sight) to measure the optic cup
- green to look for haemorrhages (red appears as much darker).

COMMON MISTAKES

- Second focus ring, with choices 0, +20 and −20, is not set to 0.
- Incorrect beam is chosen, or selection ring is left between two selections.
- Dust cover is not removed.
- Batteries are flat (most common problem).

WHAT TO DO

- Turn off the lights or draw the curtains.
- Sit opposite the patient.
- Check the focus is set at zero, and that the light works and is on the correct beam.
- Ask the patient to look at a particular point in the distance at his eye level (e.g. a light switch, a spot on the wall).

To examine the right eye (Fig. 8.2):

- Take the ophthalmoscope in your right hand.
- Approach the patient's right side.

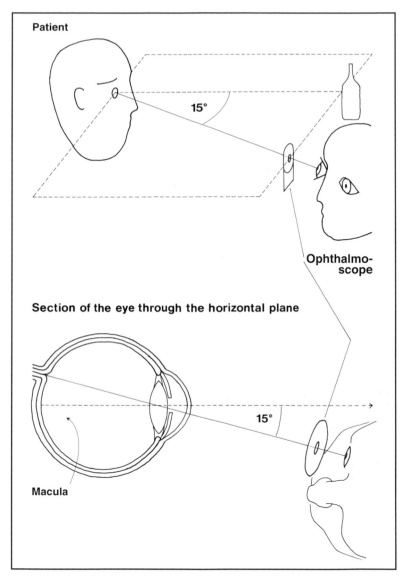

Patient

15°

**Ophthalmo-
scope**

Section of the eye through the horizontal plane

15°

Macula

Figure 8.2
Approaching the patient with an ophthalmoscope

- Look at his right eye from about 30 cm away with the ophthalmoscope in the same horizontal plane as his eye, about 15 degrees from the line of fixation. Aim at the centre of the back of his head. Keep out of the line of sight of the other eye.

- The pupil should appear pink, as in bad flash photographs. This is the red reflex.
- Opacities in the eye, notably cataracts and floaters, appear as silhouettes. Cataracts usually have a fine web-like appearance.
- Gradually move in towards the eye.
- Stay in the same horizontal plane, aiming at the back of the patient's head. This should bring you in at about 15 degrees to his line of fixation.
- Encourage the patient to keep looking at the distant point and not at the light.
- Bring the ophthalmoscope to within 1–2 cm of the eye.
- Keep the ophthalmoscope at the same level as the patient's eye and the fixation point.
- Focus the ophthalmoscope as described above.

If the eye is approached as described, the optic disc should be in view. If it is not, focus on a blood vessel and follow it. The acute angles of the branches and convergence of artery and vein indicate the direction to follow. Alternatively, start again.

 TIP   It is essential to keep the patient's eye, the point of fixation and the ophthalmoscope in the same plane.

COMMON MISTAKES

Aphakic eye (no lens): severely hypermetropic—use a high positive lens or examine while the patient has glasses on.

To examine the left eye:

Hold the ophthalmoscope in the left hand and use your left eye. If you use your right eye to look at the patient's left eye, you will end up rubbing noses with the patient. Most people find this part of the examination difficult at first so you must persevere.

1. Look at the optic disc

- Note colour.
- Look at disc margin. Is it clearly seen?
- Look at the optic cup.

2. Look at the blood vessels

Arteries (light-coloured) should be two-thirds the diameter of veins (burgundy-coloured).

- Look at the diameter of the arteries.
- Look at arteriovenous junctions.

- Look at the pattern of vessels.
- Look at the retinal veins as they turn into the optic disc and see if they pulsate, going from convex to concave. This is best appreciated as you look along the length of a vein as it runs into the optic cup.

3. Look at the retinal background

- Look adjacent to the blood vessels.
- Look at all four quadrants systematically.

WHAT YOU FIND

1. Optic disc

See Figures 8.3 and 8.4.

The optic cup is slightly on the nasal side of the centre of the optic disc. Its diameter is normally less than 50% of the disc (Figs 8.5A and 8.6).

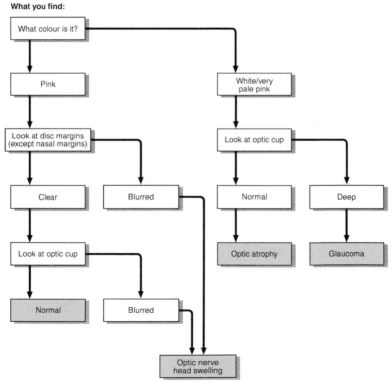

Figure 8.3
Flow chart: optic disc abnormalities

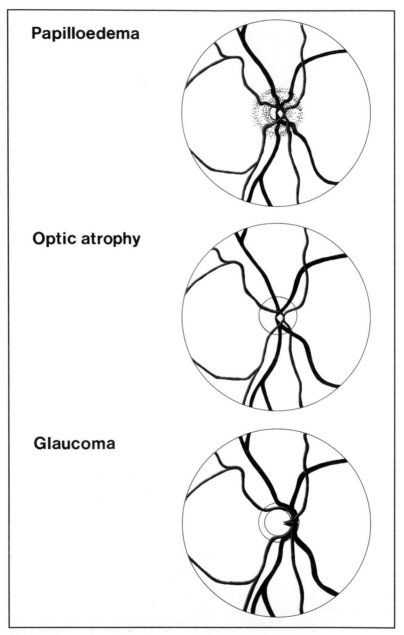

Figure 8.4
Optic disc abnormalities

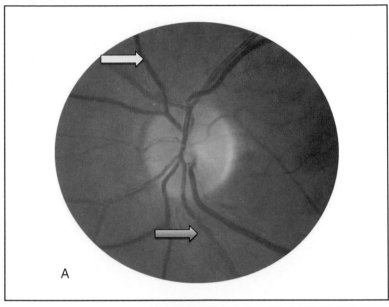

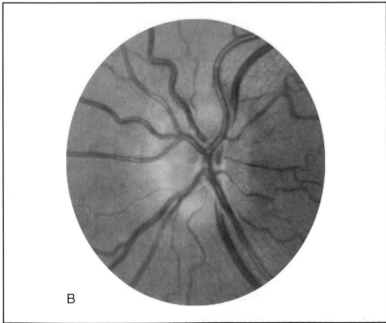

Figure 8.5
A. Normal disc, Blue arrow = artery; yellow arrow = vein; **B.** Papilloedema;
(Continued)

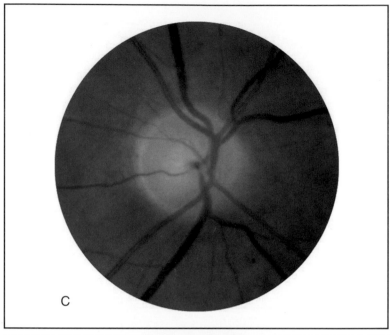

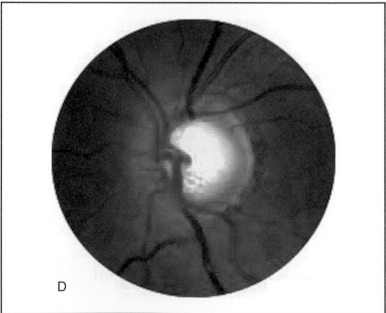

Figure 8.5, cont'd
C. Optic atrophy, note pale disc; **D.** Glaucoma, note wide optic cup.

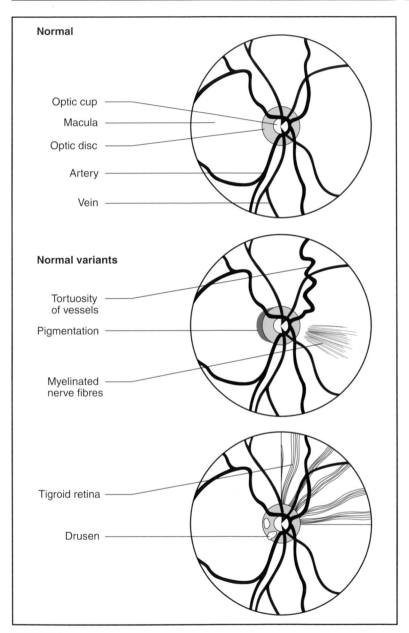

Figure 8.6
Normal variants

The optic nerve head is swollen (Fig. 8.5B). This can be caused by papilloedema or papillitis. Papilloedema usually produces more swelling, with humping of the disc margins—not usually associated with visual disturbance (may enlarge blind spot). Papillitis is associated with visual loss, especially central scotomas.

A swollen optic disc is often difficult to find, the vessels disappearing without an obvious optic disc.

The difference between papilloedema and papillitis can be remembered as follows:

- You see nothing (cannot find the disc) + patient sees everything (normal vision) = *papilloedema*.
- You see nothing + patient sees nothing (severe visual loss) = *papillitis*.
- You see everything (normal-looking disc) + patient sees nothing = *retrobulbar neuritis*.

The optic nerve head is very pale—optic atrophy (Fig. 8.5C). The optic cup is markedly enlarged, taking up most of the disc - glaucoma (Fig. 8.5D).

COMMON MISTAKES

- *Blurred nasal margin*: normal, often mistaken for papilloedema.
- *Temporal pallor*: normally paler than nasal, often misinterpreted as abnormal.
- *Myopic fundus*: myopic eye is large, so disc appears paler, may be mistaken for optic atrophy.
- *Hypermetropic fundus*: small eye, fundus appears crowded, mistaken for papilloedema.
- *Drusen*: colloid bodies that may occur on disc, mistaken for papilloedema.
- *Pigmentation on disc edge*: normal—may make disc seem pale.
- *Myelinated nerve fibres*: opaque white fibres usually radiating from disc, may be mistaken for papilloedema.

2. Blood vessels

- Irregular arterial calibre.
- Arteriovenous nipping: the vein narrows markedly as it is crossed by the artery.
- Neovascularisation: new vessels appear as fine frond-like vessels, often near the disc, frequently coming off the plane of the retina— and therefore may be out of focus.
- Bright yellow object within lumen of artery: cholesterol embolus.
- Retinal vein seen to pulsate = retinal venous pulsation present.

COMMON MISTAKES

(See Fig. 8.6)
- *Choroidal artery*: a small vessel running from disc edge towards macula. Mistaken for new vessels.
- *Tortuous vessels*: normal.

3. Retinal background (Fig. 8.7)

General background
- **Pigmented background**: normal, especially in dark-skinned people. If striped, this is called tigroid.
- **Pale**:
  - *Clear*: normal in fair-skinned people, also seen in albinos.
  - *Cloudy*: macula appears as 'cherry-red' spot, vessels narrow—seen in retinal artery occlusion.

Red lesions
- **Dot haemorrhages**: microaneurysms seen adjacent to blood vessels.
- **Blot haemorrhages**: bleeds in the deep layer of the retina from microaneurysms. Dots and blots are seen in diabetic retinopathy.
- **Flame haemorrhages**: superficial bleed shaped by nerve fibres into a fan with point towards the disc. Seen in hypertensive retinopathy; florid haemorrhages are seen in retinal venous thrombosis—may be in only one-quarter or half of the retina.
- **Subhyaloid haemorrhages**: irregular superficial haemorrhages usually with a flat top. Seen in subarachnoid haemorrhages.

White/yellow lesions
- **Hard exudates**: yellowish sharp-edged lesions. May form a ring around the macula: *macular star*. Seen in diabetes and hypertension.
- **Cotton wool spots**: white fluffy spots, sometimes also called soft exudates, caused by retinal infarcts. Seen in diabetes, systemic lupus erythematosus and acquired immunodeficiency syndrome (AIDS).

Black lesions
- **Moles**: flat, usually rounded lesions—*normal.*
- **Laser burns**: black-edged round lesions, usually in a regular pattern. Often mistaken for retinitis pigmentosa.
- **Retinitis pigmentosa**: rare, black lesions like bone spicules in the periphery of the retina.
- **Melanoma**: raised irregular malignant tumour.

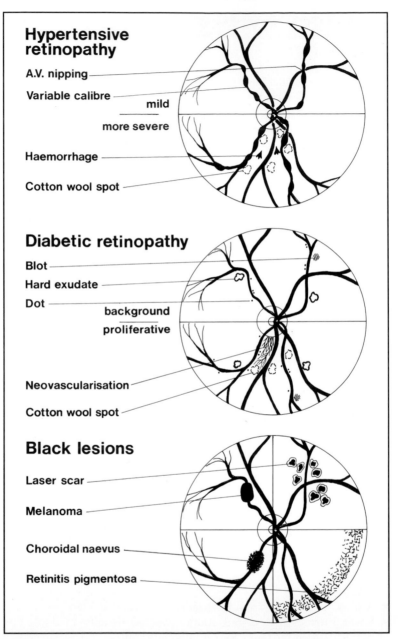

Figure 8.7
Retinal abnormalities

WHAT IT MEANS

1. Optic disc

- **Retinal venous pulsation** present: indicates normal intracranial pressure, so when it is seen it is very helpful. Retinal venous pulsation is absent in 15% of normal people, so an absence may be normal or reflect raised intracranial pressure.
- **Papilloedema.** *Common cause*: raised intracranial pressure (N.B. Absence does not exclude this). *Rarer causes*: malignant hypertension, hypercapnia.
- **Papillitis.** *Common causes*: multiple sclerosis, idiopathic.
- Optic atrophy:
  - Primary. *Common causes*: multiple sclerosis, optic nerve compression, optic nerve ischaemia. *Rarely*: nutritional deficiencies, B_{12}, B_1, hereditary.
  - Secondary: following papilloedema.
- **Deep optic cup**: chronic glaucoma—commonly idiopathic.

2. Blood vessels and retinal background

- Hypertensive retinopathy (Figs 8.7 and 8.8A&B):
  - *Stage I*: arteriolar narrowing and vessel irregularity.
  - *Stage II*: arteriovenous nipping.
  - *Stage III*: flame-shaped haemorrhages, hard exudates and cotton wool spots.
  - *Stage IV*: papilloedema.
- Diabetic retinopathy (Figs 8.7 and 8.8C&D):
  - *Background*: microaneurysms, dot and blot haemorrhages, hard exudates.
  - *Proliferative*: cotton wool spots and neovascularisation.
- Cholesterol emboli: unilateral proximal atherosclerotic lesion— usually internal carotid or common carotid stenosis.

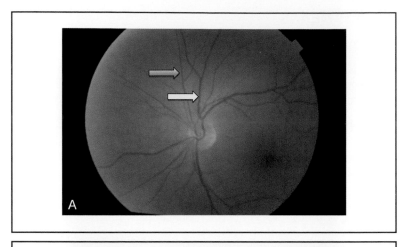

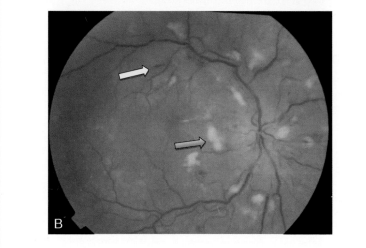

Figure 8.8
A. Normal retina: blue arrow = artery; yellow arrow = vein
B. Severe hypertensive retinopathy: blue arrow = cotton wool spot; yellow
arrow = flame haemorrhage

(Continued)

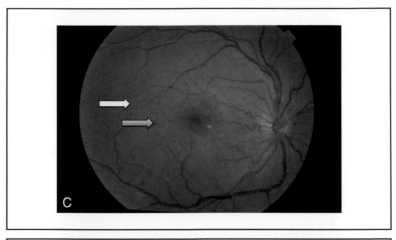

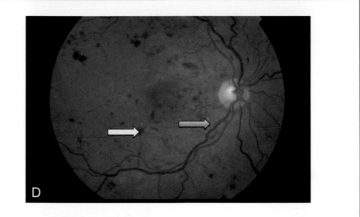

Figure 8.8, cont'd
C. Background diabetic retinopathy: blue arrow = blot haemorrhage; yellow arrow = dot haemorrhage
D. Severe diabetic retinopathy: blue arrow = hard exudate; yellow arrow = blot haemorrhage

CRANIAL NERVES III, IV, VI: **9**

EYE MOVEMENTS

BACKGROUND

Eye movements can be divided into four types:

- **Saccadic eye movements**: the rapid movement from one point of fixation to another. You would use a saccadic eye movement to look from the page to someone in the room or if you were told to look up.
- **Pursuit eye movements**: the slow eye movement used to maintain fixation on a moving object: for example, to maintain eye contact as a person moves across a room.
- **Vestibular–positional (vestibulo-ocular reflex) eye movements**: the eye movements that compensate for movement of the head to maintain fixation.
- **Convergence**: the movements that maintain fixation as an object is brought close to the face. These are rarely affected in clinical practice.

The sites of control of these eye movements differ (Fig. 9.1).

Type of eye movement	Site of control
Saccadic (command)	Frontal lobe
Pursuit	Occipital lobe
Vestibular–positional	Cerebellar vestibular nuclei
Convergence	Midbrain

In the brainstem, the inputs from the frontal and occipital lobes, the cerebellum and the vestibular nuclei are integrated so that both eyes move together. Important structures are the centre for lateral gaze in the pons and the medial longitudinal fasciculus (MLF), which runs between the nuclei of the III and IV cranial nerves (in the midbrain) and the VI (in the pons).

    The III, IV and VI cranial nerves then control the following muscles (Fig. 9.2):

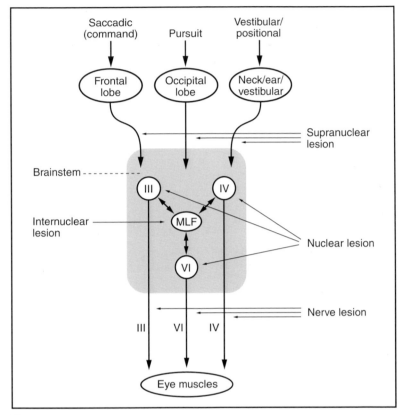

Figure 9.1
Control of eye movements

- VI: lateral rectus only
- IV: superior oblique only (SO4)
- III: the others.

Abnormalities can arise at any level (Fig. 9.1):

No double vision (generally):
- Supranuclear (above the nuclei).
- Internuclear (connections between nuclei; MLF).
- Nuclear.

Double vision:
- Nerve.
- Neuromuscular junction.
- Muscle.

Internuclear and supranuclear lesions rarely cause double vision.

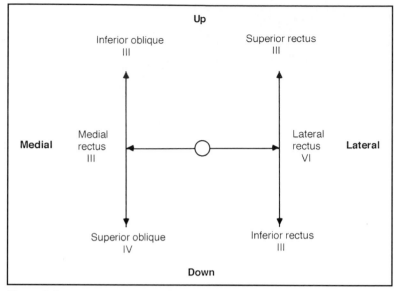

Figure 9.2
Muscles involved in eye movement

Double vision rules

- Double vision is maximal in the direction of gaze of the affected muscle.
- False image is the outer image.
- False image arises in the affected eye.

WHAT TO DO

Look at the position of the head.

- The head is tilted away from the side of a fourth nerve lesion.

Look at the eyes.

- Note ptosis (see Chapter 6).
- Note the resting position of the eyes and the position of primary gaze.

Look at the position of the eyes in primary gaze.

- Do they diverge or converge?
- Does one appear to be looking up or down—skew deviation?

Perform the cover test (Fig. 9.3).

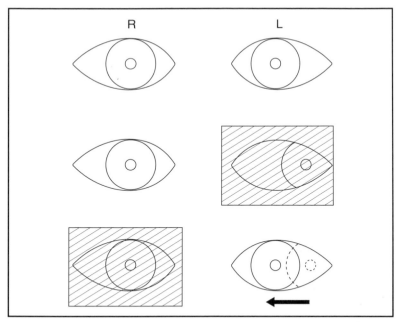

Figure 9.3
The cover test. For an explanation, see text

The cover test

What to do
This is a test for latent squint.

Ask the patient to look with both eyes at your right eye, then cover his left eye. Then uncover the left eye rapidly and cover the right eye. Look to see if the left eye has to correct to look back at your eye. Repeat, covering the left eye and watching the right eye.

What you find
If one eye has to correct as it is uncovered, this indicates that the patient has a latent strabismus (squint), which can be classified as divergent or convergent.

What it means
• **Latent squint**: congenital squint usually in the weaker eye (and myopia in childhood)—common.

Test the eye movements to pursuit

- Hold a pen vertically about 50 cm away from the patient in the centre of his gaze. Ask him to follow it with his eyes without moving his head and to tell you if he sees double. You can hold the chin lightly to prevent head movement.
- Move the pen slowly. Ask the patient to tell you if he sees double:
  - from side to side
  - up and down from the centre
  - up and down at the extreme of lateral gaze.
- Ensure the patient's nose does not prevent the pen being seen at the extreme of lateral gaze.

COMMON MISTAKES

- The target is too close.
- The target is moved too fast.
- The patient is allowed to move his head.
- In a patient with a hemianopia the target may disappear from the patient's view if moved too fast towards the hemianopia. Thus, in the presence of a hemianopia the target must be moved very slowly.

As you do this, watch the movements of the eyes.

- Do both eyes move through the full range? Estimate the percentage reduction in movement in each direction.
- Do the eyes move smoothly?
- Do both eyes move together?
- Look for nystagmus (see next chapter).

If the patient reports seeing double at any stage:

- Establish if the images are side by side, up and down, or at an angle.
- Establish the direction in which the images are widest apart.
- In this position, briefly cover one eye and ask which image disappears: the inner or outer. Repeat this by covering the other eye (Fig. 9.4).

Test saccadic eye movements

- Face the patient. Hold both your hands out in front of you about 30 cm apart from side to side and about 30 cm in front of the patient.
- Ask the patient to look from one hand to the other.
- Observe the eye movements: are they full, do they move smoothly, do they move together?
- Look particularly at the speed of adduction.

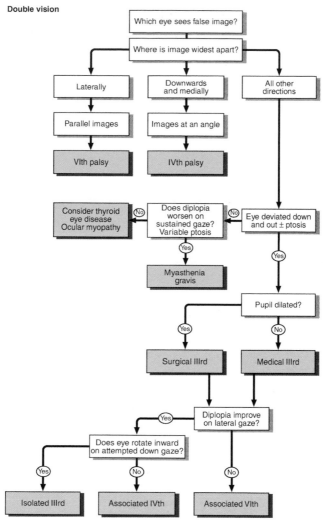

Figure 9.4
Flow chart: double vision

- Then put your hands vertically one above the other, about 30 cm apart and ask the patient to look from one to the other.
- Again observe the eye movements. Do the eyes move at a normal speed and through the full range?

Test convergence

Ask the patient to look into the distance and then look at your finger placed 50 cm in front of him. Gradually bring the eyes in, observing the limit of convergence of the eyes.

Vestibulo-ocular reflex (doll's eye manœuvre)

This test is most commonly used in unconscious patients, when it provides a way of testing eye movements. In conscious patients with limited eye movements on command or pursuit, the test can be used to demonstrate preserved eye movements on vestibulo-positional stimulation, indicating a supranuclear eye movement abnormality.

Ask the patient to look into the distance at a fixed point; turn his head to the left then the right, and flex the neck and extend the neck.

The eyes should move within the orbits, maintaining forward gaze.

WHAT YOU FIND

- **The eyes are misaligned** in primary gaze:
  - The misalignment remains *constant* in all directions for gaze = convergent or divergent concomitant strabismus (squint).
  - *One eye is deviated* downwards and out, with ptosis = third nerve lesion.
  - Eyes aligned in different vertical planes = skew deviation.
- The patient has double vision (Fig. 9.4):

  Try to answer the following questions:
  Is there a single nerve (VI, III or IV) deficit (Fig. 9.5)?

  - If there is a third nerve deficit, is it medical (pupil-sparing) or surgical (with pupillary dilatation)?

  If not single nerve:

  - Is there a combination of single nerves?
  - Is it myasthenia or dysthyroid eye disease?
- The patient does not have double vision: Compare movements on command, on pursuit and on vestibular positional testing.

Other common abnormalities:

- Patient does not look towards one side = lateral gaze palsy; check response to vestibulo-ocular reflex testing (Fig. 9.6).
- Patient does not look up = upgaze palsy.
- Patient does not look down = downgaze palsy.
- Eyes do not move together, with markedly slowed adduction and with nystagmus in the abducting eye = internuclear ophthalmoplegia with ataxic nystagmus (Fig. 9.7).
- Eye movement falls short of target and requires a second movement to fixate = hypometric saccades.

Rarer abnormalities:

- Loss to command only = frontal lesion.
- Loss to pursuit only = occipital lesion.
- Limited eye movements on command or pursuit with normal movements on vestibulo-ocular reflex = supranuclear palsy.

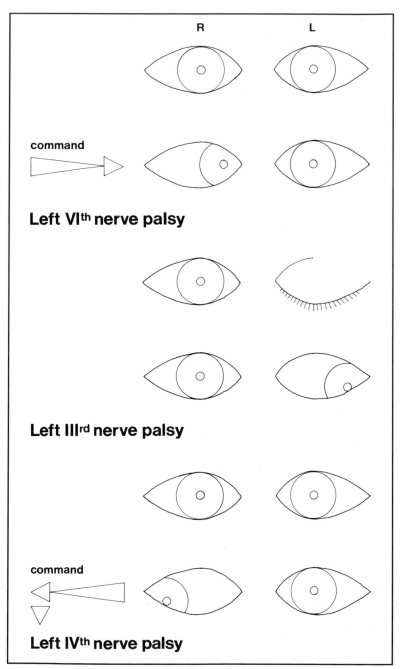

Figure 9.5
Single nerve palsies

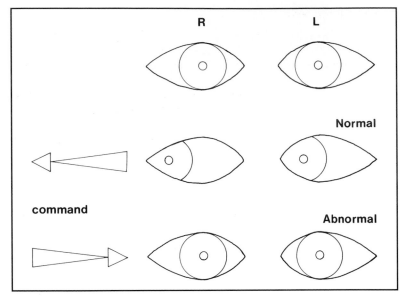

Figure 9.6
Left lateral gaze palsy

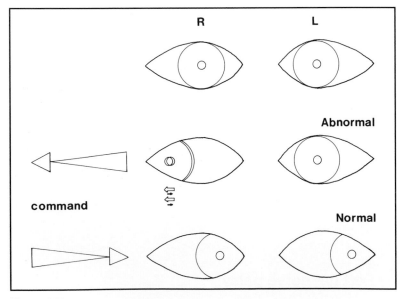

Figure 9.7
Left internuclear ophthalmoplegia. There is nystagmus of the right eye as the eye looks to the right

WHAT IT MEANS

- **Skew deviation**: brainstem lesion. *Common causes*: stroke, demyelination—look for associated brainstem signs.
- **Single cranial nerve palsy (III, IV or VI)**: lesion along the course of the nerve or a nuclear lesion. *Common causes*:
  - *Medical*: diabetes mellitus, atherosclerosis. *Rarely*: vasculitis, Miller–Fisher syndrome (a form of Guillain–Barré syndrome).
  - *Surgical* (N.B. pupil involvement in third nerve palsy): tumour, aneurysm, trauma, a false localising sign or uncal herniation (third nerve).

 TIP   Posterior communicating aneurysm is a common cause of a surgical third nerve palsy.

- **Nuclear lesions**: arise from brainstem pathology, including brainstem infarction, multiple sclerosis and, rarely, brainstem haemorrhage and tumour.
- **Lateral gaze palsy**: can arise from:
  - a large frontal or parietal lobe lesion when the patient looks away from the paralysed side (can be overcome by doll's eye manoeuvre)
  - a pontine lesion when the patient cannot look to the non-paralysed side and there may be other pontine abnormalities (facial weakness); not overcome using doll's eye manoeuvre.
- **Vertical gaze palsy**: lesions in the upper brainstem.

  Common causes of lateral and vertical gaze palsies: brainstem infarction, multiple sclerosis, tumour.

- **Internuclear ophthalmoplegia** = a lesion to the medial longitudinal fasciculus. *Common cause*: multiple sclerosis. *Rarer causes*: vascular disease, pontine glioma.
- **Supranuclear palsy** with preserved positional/vestibular testing: may arise in association with akinetic rigid syndromes (Chapter 24), when it is referred to as the *Steele–Richardson syndrome* or *progressive supranuclear palsy*, and may be seen in other degenerative conditions.
- **Hypometric saccades**: indicate a cerebellar lesion—see Chapter 23.

CRANIAL NERVES: 10

NYSTAGMUS

BACKGROUND

Nystagmus is an oscillation of the eyes. This can be a symmetrical oscillation—pendular nystagmus—or faster in one direction—jerk nystagmus. In jerk nystagmus there is a slow drift in one direction with a fast correction in the opposite direction. It is conventional to describe the nystagmus in the direction of the fast phase. If the oscillation is a twisting movement, this is torsional or rotatory nystagmus.

Nystagmus can be:

- *physiological*: oculokinetic nystagmus (as seen in people looking out of the windows of trains)
- *peripheral*: due to abnormalities of the vestibular system in the ear, the eighth nerve nucleus or the nerve itself
- *central*: due to abnormalities of the central vestibular connections or cerebellum
- *retinal*: due to the inability to fixate.

WHAT TO DO

Ask the patient to follow your finger with both eyes. Move the finger in turn up, down and to each side. Hold the finger briefly in each position at a point where the finger can easily be seen by both eyes.

Watch for nystagmus. Note:

- whether it is symmetrical, moving at the same speed in both directions (*pendular nystagmus*), or if there is a fast phase in one direction with a slow phase in the other (*jerk nystagmus*)
- the direction of the fast phase—is it in the horizontal plane, in the vertical plane or rotatory?
- the position of the eye when nystagmus occurs and when it is most marked
- whether it occurs only towards the direction of gaze (*first degree*), in the primary position of gaze (*second degree*) and whether it occurs with the fast phase going away from the direction of gaze (*third degree*)

- whether it affects the abducting eye more than the adducting eye
- whether it occurs in one direction only
- whether it occurs in the direction of gaze in more than one direction (*multidirectional gaze-evoked nystagmus*).

To decide whether it is central or peripheral, note:

- whether it persists or fatigues
- whether it is associated with a feeling of vertigo
- whether it improves with visual fixation.

COMMON MISTAKES

- At the extreme of lateral gaze, one or two nystagmoid jerks can be seen normally, especially if the target is too close—ensure that the target remains within binocular vision.
- If nystagmoid jerks are found, repeat the test. If this is true nystagmus, it will appear at less than extreme lateral gaze.

Special test: optokinetic nystagmus (OKN)

This can be tested when a striped drum is spun in front of the eyes; this normally evokes nystagmus in the opposite direction to the direction of spin. This is a useful test for patients with hysterical blindness.

Tests for benign positional vertigo are described in Chapter 12.

WHAT YOU FIND

See Figure 10.1.

Decide whether central or peripheral.

Central versus peripheral nystagmus

	Sustained	Fatigue	Associated with symptoms of vertigo	Reduced by fixation
Central	+	−	−	−
Peripheral	−	+	+	+

Peripheral nystagmus is not associated with other eye movement abnormalities and usually has a rotatory component.

WHAT IT MEANS

- **Nystagmoid jerks**: normal.
- **Pendular nystagmus**: inability to fixate—congenital; occurs with albinisim and blindness and may occur in miners.

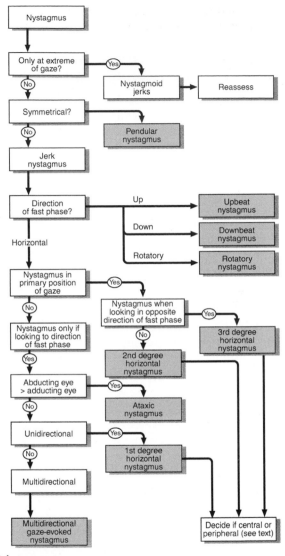

Figure 10.1
Flow chart: nystagmus

- Rotatory (or rotary) nystagmus:
  - *Pure* rotatory nystagmus = central; peripheral horizontal nystagmus usually has a rotatory component.
- **Vertical nystagmus** (rare): indicates brainstem disease.
  - *Upbeat*: indicates upper brainstem. *Common causes*: demyelination, stroke, Wernicke's encephalopathy.

- *Downbeat*: indicates medullary–cervical junction lesion. *Common causes*: Arnold–Chiari malformation, syringobulbia, demyelination.
- Horizontal nystagmus (common):
  - **Ataxic nystagmus**: nystagmus of abducting eye >>adducting eye, associated with internuclear ophthalmoplegia (see Chapter 9). *Common causes*: multiple sclerosis, cerebrovascular disease.
  - **Multidirectional gaze-evoked nystagmus**: nystagmus in the direction of gaze, occurring in more than one direction. Always central—cerebellar or vestibular. Cerebellar syndrome. *Common causes*: drugs, alcohol, multiple sclerosis. *Rarer causes*: cerebellar degeneration, cerebellar tumours.
  - *Central vestibular syndromes. Common causes*: younger patients—multiple sclerosis; older patients—vascular disease.
  - **Unidirectional nystagmus**: second- and third-degree horizontal nystagmus is usually central; if peripheral it must be acute and associated with severe vertigo. First-degree horizontal nystagmus may be central or peripheral:
  peripheral:
  - **peripheral vestibular syndromes.** *Common causes*: vestibular neuronitis, Ménière's disease, vascular lesions
  central:
  - **unilateral cerebellar syndrome.** *Common causes*: as central vestibular syndromes. *Rarer causes*: tumour or abscess
  - **unilateral central vestibular syndrome.** *Common causes*: as central vestibular syndromes.
- Unusual and rare eye movement abnormalities:
  - **Opsoclonus**: rapid oscillations of the eyes in the horizontal rotatory or vertical direction—indicates brainstem disease, site uncertain, often a paraneoplastic syndrome
  - **Ocular bobbing**: eyes drifting up and down in the vertical plane—associated with pontine lesions.

CRANIAL NERVES V AND VII:

11

THE FACE

BACKGROUND

Facial nerve: VII

Peripheral function can be summarised as 'face, ear, taste, tear':

- *face*: muscles of facial expression and blinking
- *ear*: stapedius (the muscle that dampens loud noises) and sensory supply to the external auditory meatus and adjacent pinna.
- *taste*: anterior two-thirds of the tongue
- *tear*: parasympathetic supply to the lacrimal glands.

With **lower motor neurone (LMN) facial weakness,** all muscles are affected.

With **upper motor neurone (UMN) facial weakness,** the forehead is relatively preserved.

Trigeminal nerve: V

Sensory

There are three divisions:

- ophthalmic (V_1)
- maxillary (V_2)
- mandibular (V_3).

For distribution, see Figure 11.1. V_1 supplies the cornea.

Motor

The trigeminal nerve supplies the muscles of mastication.

What to do

Look at the face generally.

- Is there a general medical syndrome (e.g. hyper- or hypothyroidism, Cushing's disease, acromegaly or Paget's disease)?
- Is the face motionless?
- Are there abnormal movements (see Chapter 24)?

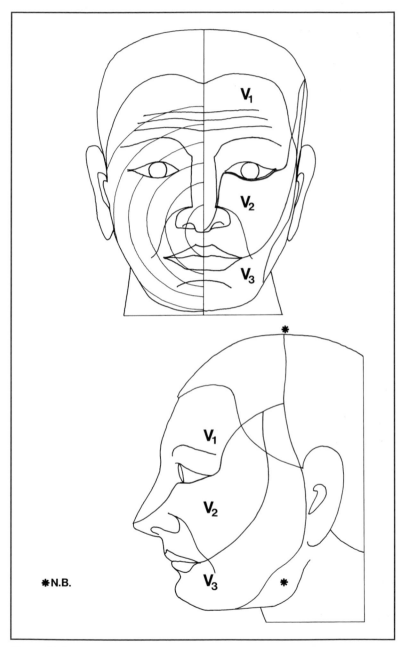

Figure 11.1
Facial sensation. *Left side*: ophthalmic (V$_1$), maxillary (V$_2$) and mandibular (V$_3$)
divisions of the trigeminal nerve. *Right side*: muzzle pattern of innervation. Rings
further from the nose go further down the brainstem. *N.B. The angle of the jaw is
not supplied by the trigeminal nerve

FACIAL NERVE: WHAT TO DO

Look at the symmetry of the face.

- Note nasolabial folds and forehead wrinkles (Fig. 11.2).
- Watch spontaneous movements: smiling, blinking.

Ask the patient to:

- **show you his teeth** (*demonstrate*)
- **whistle**
- **close his eyes tightly** as if he had soap in them (*demonstrate*)
  - watch eye movement
  - assess the strength by trying to open his eyes with your fingers
- look up at the ceiling.

Look out for symmetrical movement.

Compare the strength of the forehead and lower face.

In LMN lesions you can see the eye turn upwards on attempted closure—*Bell's phenomenon*.

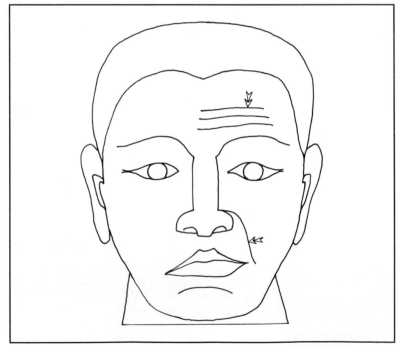

Figure 11.2
Right-sided lower motor neurone VII. Note absent facial lines and droopy mouth

> ## COMMON MISTAKES
>
> - *Mild facial asymmetry without weakness*: normal. Ask the patient to look in a mirror.
> - Ptosis is *not* due to weakness of muscles supplied by VII.

Other functions of the facial nerve

Look at the external auditory meatus—the cutaneous distribution of VII. Note any vesicles suggestive of herpes zoster.

Provides taste to the anterior two-thirds of tongue. Taste is rarely tested and requires saline solution and sugar solution. A cotton bud is dipped in the solution and applied to the tongue and the patient is asked to identify it. Test each side of the anterior two-thirds and the posterior one-third.

FACIAL NERVE: WHAT YOU FIND

See Figure 11.3.

Bilateral facial nerve weakness can be easily missed unless tested for. Think of it if you feel that a patient seems impassive when you talk to him. He may not be depressed; his face might not be able to move!

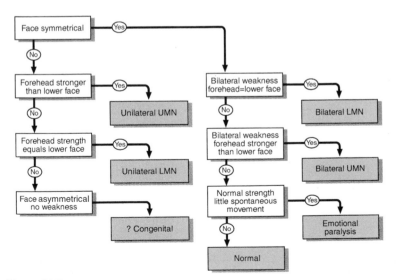

Figure 11.3
Flow chart: facial nerve abnormalities

Failure of the patient to smile when asked to whistle has been noted in patients with emotional paralysis due to parkinsonism: the 'whistle–smile' sign.

FACIAL NERVE: WHAT IT MEANS

- **Unilateral LMN weakness**: lesion of the facial nerve or its nucleus in the pons. *Common cause*: Bell's palsy. *More rarely*: pontine vascular accidents, lesions at the cerebellopontine angle, herpetic infections (Ramsay Hunt syndrome—note vesicles in external auditory meatus), Lyme disease, basal meningitis, lesions in its course through the temporal bone, parotid tumours.
- **Bilateral LMN weakness**: *Common causes*: sarcoidosis, Guillain–Barré syndrome. *Rarer causes*: myasthenia gravis can produce bilateral fatigable facial weakness (neuromuscular junction); myopathies can produce bilateral facial weakness (N.B. myotonic dystrophy and fascio-scapulo-humeral dystrophy).
- **Unilateral UMN**: cerebrovascular accidents, demyelination, tumours—may be associated with ipsilateral hemiplegia (supratentorial lesions) or contralateral hemiplegia (brainstem lesions).
- **Bilateral UMN**: pseudobulbar palsy, motor neurone disease.
- **Emotional paralysis**: parkinsonism.

TRIGEMINAL NERVE: WHAT TO DO

Motor

Test muscles of mastication (trigeminal nerve: motor)
Look at the side of the face.

- Is there wasting of the temporalis muscle?

Ask the patient to clench his teeth.

- Feel the masseter and temporalis muscles.

Ask the patient to push his mouth open against your hand.

- Resist his jaw opening with your hand under his chin. Note if the jaw deviates to one side.

Jaw jerk.

- Ask the patient to let his mouth hang loosely open. Place your finger on his chin. Percuss your finger with the patella hammer. Feel and observe the jaw movement.

Sensory

Test facial sensation (trigeminal nerve: sensory). (See Chapter 19 for general comments on sensory testing.)

Test light touch and pinprick in each division on both sides:

- V_1: forehead
- V_2: cheek
- V_3: lower lip (Fig. 11.1).

Compare one side to the other.

- *If abnormal*, test temperature.
- *If a sensory deficit is found,* determine its edges, moving from abnormal to normal.

THE CORNEAL REFLEX (AFFERENT— OPHTHALMIC BRANCH OF V; EFFERENT—VII)

- Ask the patient to look up and away from you. Bring a piece of cotton wool twisted to a point to touch the cornea from the side.
- Watch both eyes blink closed.
- If there is a unilateral facial palsy, the sensation of the cornea can be demonstrated if the opposite eye is watched.

COMMON MISTAKES

- The conjunctiva is touched instead of the cornea (Fig. 11.4).
- Reflex is mildly inhibited in contact lens wearers.
- Cotton wool brought in too quickly acts as a menacing stimulus to provoke a blink.

Following corneal stimulation

- Failure of either side of face to contract = V_1 lesion
- Failure of only one side to contract = VII lesion
- Subjective reduction in corneal sensation = partial V_1

An absent corneal reflex can be an early and objective sign of sensory trigeminal lesion.

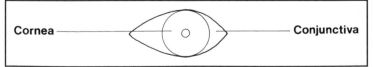

Cornea ———————————⟨ ○ ⟩——————————— Conjunctiva

Figure 11.4
Corneal reflex: touch the cornea!

TRIGEMINAL NERVE: WHAT YOU FIND

Motor

- Wasting of temporalis and masseter: rare. *Causes*: myotonic dystrophy, motor neurone disease, fascio-scapulo-humeral dystrophy.
- Weakness of jaw closure: very rare.
- Weakness of jaw opening: jaw deviates to the side of the lesion. *Cause*: unilateral lesion of motor V.

Jaw jerk

- No movement: *absent jaw jerk.*
- Minimal movement: *present normal jaw jerk.*
- Brisk movement: *brisk jaw jerk.*

Sensory

- *Impairment or loss in one or more divisions on one side* (Fig. 11.1): of light touch or pinprick and temperature or both.
- *Unilateral facial loss*: one or all modalities.
- Muzzle loss of pinprick and temperature.
- *Unilateral area of sensory loss* not in distribution of whole division.
- *Trigger zone that produces facial pain.*

N.B.

- Angle of jaw is not supplied by the trigeminal but by the greater auricular (C2).
- The trigeminal innervates the scalp to the vertex not just to the hairline.

TRIGEMINAL NERVE: WHAT IT MEANS

- Loss of all modalities in one or more divisions:
  - *Lesion in sensory ganglion*: most commonly herpes zoster.
  - *Lesion of division during intracranial course*: V_1 cavernous sinus (associated III, IV, VI) or orbital fissure, V_2 trauma, V_3 basal tumours (usually associated motor V).
- Loss of sensation in all divisions in all modalities:
  - Lesion of the Gasserian ganglion, sensory root or sensory nucleus: lesions of cerebellopontine angle (associated VII, VIII), basal meningitis (e.g. sarcoid, carcinoma); trigeminal sensory neuropathy can occur in Sjogren's syndrome.
- Loss of light touch only:
  - With ipsilateral hemisensory loss of light touch: contralateral parietal lobe lesion.
  - With no other loss: sensory root lesion in pons.

- Loss of pinprick and temperature with associated contralateral loss of these modalities on the body: ipsilateral brainstem lesion.
- Loss of sensation in muzzle distribution: lesion of descending spinal sensory nucleus with lowest level outermost—syringomyelia, demyelination.
- Area of sensory loss on cheek or lower jaw: damage to branches of V_2 or V_3 infiltration by metastases.
- Trigger area: trigeminal neuralgia.

CRANIAL NERVE VIII: 12

AUDITORY NERVE

There are two components: auditory and vestibular.

AUDITORY

WHAT TO DO

Test the hearing

Test one ear at a time. Block the opposite ear; either cover it with your hand or produce a blocking white noise, e.g. crumpling paper.

Hold your watch by the patient's ear. Discover how far away from the ear it is still heard. Alternative sounds are whispering or rubbing your fingers together. Increase in volume to normal speech or loud speech until your patient hears.

If the hearing in one ear is reduced, perform Rinne's and Weber's tests.

Rinne's test
- Hold a 256 or 512 Hz tuning fork on the mastoid process (bone conduction (BC)) and then in the front of the ear (air conduction (AC)).
- Ask the patient in which position the sound is louder.

Weber's test
- Hold the 256 or 512 Hz tuning fork on the vertex of the head.
- Ask in which ear the sound is louder: the good ear or the deaf ear.

WHAT YOU FIND

	Rinne test in deaf ear	Weber test
Conductive deafness	BC > AC	Deaf ear
Sensorineural deafness	AC > BC	Good ear

N.B. With complete sensorineural deafness in one ear, bone conduction from the other ear will be better than air conduction.

WHAT IT MEANS

- **Conductive deafness.** *Common causes*: middle ear disease, external auditory meatus obstruction, e.g. wax.
- **Sensorineural deafness:**
  - *Lesion of the cochlea* (common): otosclerosis, Ménière's disease, drug- or noise-induced damage.
  - *Lesions in the nerve* (uncommon): meningitis, cerebellopontine angle tumours, trauma.
  - *Lesions in the nucleus in the pons* (very rare): vascular or demyelinating lesions.

VESTIBULAR

BACKGROUND

The vestibular system is not easy to examine at the bedside because it is difficult to test one part of the system, or even one side, in isolation. In some respects this is fortunate, as it is this ability of the vestibular system that allows patients to make good recoveries even after severe unilateral vestibular lesions by learning to operate on only one functioning vestibular system.

The vestibular system can be examined indirectly by checking gait, looking for nystagmus and carrying out more specific tests (see below).

Gait

See Chapter 4. Always test heel–toe walking. Gait is unsteady, veering to the side of the lesion.

Nystagmus

See Chapter 10. Vestibular nystagmus is associated with vertigo, horizontal and unidirectional. It may be positional.

Head impulse test

See Chapter 25. This is a dynamic test of vestibular function.

Caloric test

This is normally performed in a test laboratory.

The patient lies down with his head on a pillow at 30 degrees so the lateral semicircular canal is vertical.

Cool water (usually about 250 ml at 30°C) is instilled into one ear over 40 seconds. The patient is asked to look straight ahead and the eyes are watched. This is repeated in the other ear, and then in each ear with warm water (44°C).

CALORIC TESTING: WHAT YOU FIND

- Normal responses:
  - *cold water*: nystagmus fast-phase away from stimulated ear
  - *warm water*: nystagmus fast-phase towards stimulated ear.
- Reduced response to cold and warm stimuli in one ear: *canal paresis*.
- Reduced nystagmus in one direction after warm stimuli from one ear and cold stimuli from the other: *directional preponderance*.

N.B. In the unconscious patient, the normal responses are as follows:

- *cold water*: tonic movement of the eyes towards the stimulus
- *warm water*: tonic movement of the eyes away from the stimulus.

(The fast phase of nystagmus is produced by the correction of this response, which is absent in the unconscious patient.)

CALORIC TESTING: WHAT IT MEANS

- **Canal paresis**: lesion of the semicircular canal (Ménière's disease) or nerve damage (causes as for sensorineural deafness, plus vestibular neuronitis).
- **Directional preponderance**: vestibular nuclear lesions (brainstem). *Common causes*: vascular disease, demyelination.

FURTHER TESTS OF VESTIBULAR FUNCTION

Hallpike's test

This is used in patients with positional vertigo.

- Sit the patient on a flat bed so that when he lies down his head will not be supported.
- Turn the head to one side and ask the patient to look to that side.
- The patient then lies back quickly until he is flat, with his neck extended and his head supported by the examiner (Fig. 12.1).
- Watch for nystagmus in the direction of gaze. Note if this is associated with a delay, whether it fatigues when the test is repeated and if the patient feels vertigo. Repeat for the other side.

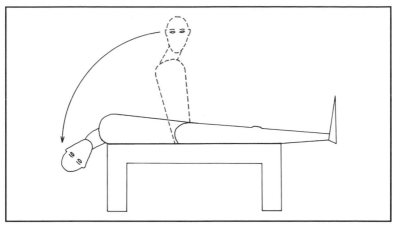

Figure 12.1
Hallpike's manœuvre

What you find and what it means
- No nystagmus: normal.
- Fatigable rotatory nystagmus with delay: peripheral vestibular syndrome, usually benign positional vertigo.
- Non-fatigable nystagmus without delay: central vestibular syndrome.

Turning test
- Ask the patient to stand facing you.
- Ask him to point both arms straight out in front of him towards you.
- Ask him to walk on the spot; when he is doing this, he should then close his eyes.
- Watch his position.

What you find and what it means
The patient gradually turns to one side, and may turn through 180 degrees. This indicates a lesion on the side he turns towards.

CRANIAL NERVES IX, X, XII: 13

THE MOUTH

BACKGROUND

Glossopharyngeal nerve: IX

- *Sensory*: posterior one-third of tongue, pharynx, middle ear.
- *Motor*: stylopharyngeus.
- *Autonomic*: to salivary glands (parotid).

Vagus nerve: X

- *Sensory*: tympanic membrane, external auditory canal and external ear.
- *Motor*: muscles of palate, pharynx, larynx (via recurrent laryngeal).
- *Autonomic*: afferents from carotid baroreceptors, parasympathetic supply to and from thorax and abdomen.

Hypoglossal nerve: XII

- *Sensory*: none.
- *Motor*: intrinsic muscles of the tongue.

MOUTH AND TONGUE: WHAT TO DO

Ask the patient to open his mouth.
Look at the gums.

- Are they hypertrophied?

Look at the tongue.

- Is it normal in size?
- Are there rippling movements (fasciculations)?
- Is it normal in colour and texture?

Ask the patient to put out his tongue.

- Does it move straight out or deviate to one side?

COMMON MISTAKES

- Small rippling movements of the tongue are normal when the tongue is protruded or held in a particular position.
- Fasciculations need to be looked for when the tongue is at rest in the mouth.

To assess weakness
Ask the patient to push his tongue into his cheek and test the power by pushing against it; repeat on both sides.

Test repeated movements
Ask the patient to put his tongue in and out as fast as he can, and move it from side to side. Look at the speed of tongue movement. Ask the patient to say 'ticker ticker ticker' as fast as he can.

Test speech
See dysarthria (Chapter 2).

MOUTH: WHAT YOU FIND AND WHAT IT MEANS

- **Gum hypertrophy**: phenytoin therapy.
- **Red, 'beefy' tongue**: vitamin B_{12} deficiency.
- **Large tongue**: amyloidosis, acromegaly, congenital hypothyroidism.
- **Saliva pooling in mouth**: indicates swallowing difficultly.
- **Small tongue**: *with fasciculations* = bilateral lower motor neurone lesion; motor neurone disease (progressive bulbar palsy type), basal meningitis, syringobulbia.
- **Small tongue**: *with reduced speed of movements* = bilateral upper motor neurone lesion—often associated with labile emotions, increased jaw jerk: pseudobulbar palsy.
- **Small tongue**: *with fasciculations and reduced speed of movements* = mixed bilateral upper and lower motor neurone lesions; motor neurone disease (progressive bulbar palsy type).
- **Tongue deviates to one side** = weakness on the side it moves towards.
  - *With unilateral wasting and fasciculation*: unilateral lower motor neurone disease (rare). *Causes*: syringomyelia, basal meningitis, early motor neurone disease, foramen magnum tumour.
  - *With normal bulk*: unilateral upper motor neurone weakness (common)—associated with hemiparesis: strokes, tumours.
- **Tongue moves in and out on protrusion ('trombone' tremor)**: cerebellar disease, essential tremor, extrapyramidal syndromes.

PHARYNX: WHAT TO DO

Look at the position of the uvula.

- Is it central?

If you cannot see the uvula, use a tongue depressor.
  Ask the patient to say 'Ahh'.
  Look at the uvula.

- Does it move up centrally?
- Does it move over to one side?

Additional testing:
If the patient is alert and co-operative and sitting up and swallowing appears safe, ask the patient to swallow (provide a glass of water).

- Watch for smooth coordination of action.
- Note:
  – if there are two phases, with a delay between the oral and pharyngeal phase or
  – if swallowing is followed by coughing or breathlessness, which suggest aspiration.

GAG REFLEX: WHAT TO DO

Afferent: glossopharyngeal nerve. *Efferent*: vagus.

- Touch the pharyngeal wall behind the pillars of the fauces (Fig. 13.1).
- Watch the uvula; it should lift following the stimulus.
- Ask the patient to compare the sensation between two sides.

PHARYNX AND GAG REFLEX: WHAT YOU FIND

- Uvula moves to one side: upper or lower motor lesion of vagus on the other side.
- Uvula does not move on saying 'ahh' or gag: bilateral palatal muscle paresis.
- Uvula moves on saying 'ahh' but not on gag, with reduced sensation of pharynx: IX palsy (rare).

LARYNX: WHAT TO DO

Ask the patient to cough.
  Listen to the onset.

- Explosive or gradual?

Listen to the speech (see Chapter 3).

- Are volume and quality normal?
- Does the speech fatigue?

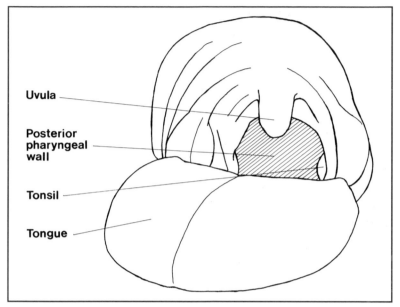

Figure 13.1
The mouth

Laryngoscopy

Direct visualisation of the vocal cords can be achieved through laryngoscopy, which allows the position of the vocal cords and their movement to be assessed. This normally requires an ENT opinion.

LARYNX: WHAT YOU FIND

- Gradual-onset cough—bovine cough: suggests *vocal cord palsy.*
- Bubbly voice and cough: suggests *combined cord palsy and pharyngeal pooling due to X nerve lesion.*
- Swallow followed by coughing indicates aspiration due to poor airway protection: suggests *X nerve lesion.*
- Unilateral cord palsy: *recurrent laryngeal palsy or vagal lesion.*

PHARYNX AND LARYNX: WHAT IT MEANS

- **Tenth nerve palsy** may be due to lesions in the medulla: look for associated ipsilateral cerebellar signs, loss of pain and temperature in the face on the same side and on the body on the opposite side, and an ipsilateral Horner's (lateral medullary syndrome).
    - Extramedullary and intracranial: look for associated XI cranial, IX cranial nerves.
    - N.B. Left-sided recurrent laryngeal palsy may arise from mediastinal or intrathoracic pathology.

- **Bilateral lower motor neurone X** occurs in progressive bulbar palsy (a variant of motor neurone disease (MND)): look for associated tongue fasciculations and mixed upper and lower motor neurone signs without sensory loss in the limbs.
- **Bilateral pharyngeal weakness and/or bilateral vocal cord weakness** can also occur in myasthenia gravis. This weakness is usually fatigable.

CRANIAL NERVE XI: 14

ACCESSORY NERVE

BACKGROUND

The spinal accessory nerve arises from the medulla and has contributions from the spinal route rising from C2 to C4. It is purely motor and innervates the sternocleidomastoid and the trapezius.

The ipsilateral cerebral hemisphere supplies the contralateral trapezius and the ipsilateral sternocleidomastoid. Thus, a single upper motor lesion can give rise to signs on both sides.

WHAT TO DO

Look at the neck.

- Is the sternocleidomastoid wasted or fasciculating?
- Is the sternocleidomastoid hypertrophied?
- Is the head position normal?

Look at the shoulders.

- Are they wasted or fasciculating?

Sternocleidomastoid
Ask the patient to lift his head forward.
Push the head back with your hand on his forehead. Look at both sternocleidomastoids.

Ask the patient to turn his head to one side.
Push against his forehead. Watch the opposite sternocleidomastoid.

Trapezius
Ask the patient to shrug his shoulders.
Watch for symmetry.
Push down the shoulders.

WHAT YOU FIND AND WHAT IT MEANS

- Weakness of sternocleidomastoid and trapezius on the same side: *peripheral accessory palsy*. Look for associated ipsilateral IX and X lesions: suggests a jugular foramen lesion (glomus tumour or neurofibroma).
- Weakness of ipsilateral sternocleidomastoid and contralateral trapezius: *upper motor neurone weakness on ipsilateral side.*
- Unilateral delayed shoulder shrug: suggests *contralateral upper motor neurone lesion.*
- Bilateral wasting and weakness of sternocleidomastoid indicates *myopathy* (such as myotonic dystrophy, fascio-scapulo-humeral dystrophy or polymyositis) or *motor neurone disease* (look for associated bulbar abnormalities).
- Unilateral sternocleidomastoid abnormalities: indicate *unilateral trauma, unilateral XI nerve weakness* or *upper motor neurone weakness* (check opposite trapezius).
- Abnormal head position and hypertrophy of neck muscles occur in *cervical dystonia* (see Chapter 24).

GENERAL

There are five patterns of muscular weakness:

1. **Upper motor neurone (UMN)**: increased tone, increased reflexes, pyramidal pattern of weakness (weak extensors in the arm, weak flexors in the leg).
2. **Lower motor neurone (LMN)**: wasting, fasciculation, decreased tone and reduced or absent reflexes.
3. **Muscle disease**: wasting, decreased tone, impaired or absent reflexes.
4. **Neuromuscular junction**: fatigable weakness, normal or decreased tone, normal reflexes.
5. **Functional weakness**: normal tone, normal reflexes without wasting with erratic power.

The level of the nervous system affected can be determined by the distribution and pattern of the weakness and by associated findings (Table 15.1).

Examples of brainstem signs (all contralateral to the upper motor neurone weakness): third, fourth and sixth palsies, seventh lower motor neurone loss, nystagmus and dysarthria.

Hemisphere signs: aphasia, visual field defects, inattention or neglect, higher function deficits.

Mixed UMN and LMN lesions: motor neurone disease (with normal sensation), or combined cervical myelopathy and radiculopathy and lumbar radiculopathy (with sensory abnormalities).

Functional weakness should be considered when:

- the weakness is not in a distribution that can be understood on an anatomical basis
- the movements are very variable and power is erratic
- there is a difference between the apparent power of moving a limb voluntarily and when power is being tested
- as long as there are no changes in tone or reflexes.

Table 15.1
Approach to weakness*

Generalised weakness (limbs and cranial nerves)	
Diffuse disease of:	
Nerve	Polyradiculopathy
Neuromuscular junction	Myasthenia gravis
Muscle	Myopathy
Weakness all four limbs	
Upper motor neurone	Cervical cord lesion
	Brainstem lesion
Lower motor neurone	Bilateral cerebral lesions
	Polyradiculopathy
Mixed upper and lower motor	Peripheral neuropathy
neurone	Motor neurone disease
Muscle	Myopathy
Unilateral and leg weakness	
Upper motor neurone	Hemisection of cervical cord
	N.B. sensory signs
	Brainstem lesion
	N.B. brainstem signs
	Cerebral lesion
	N.B. hemisphere signs
Weakness both legs	
Upper motor neurone	Spinal cord lesion
Lower motor neurone	Cauda equina lesion
	N.B. sphincter involvement
	in both
Single limb	
Upper motor neurone	Lesion above highest involved level
	N.B. other signs may help localise
Lower motor neurone	Single nerve = mononeuropathy
	Single root = radiculopathy
Patchy weakness	
Upper motor neurone	Multiple CNS lesions
Lower motor neurone	Polyradiculopathy
	Multiple single nerves = mononeuritis multiplex
Variable weakness	
Non-anatomical distribution	Consider functional weakness or myasthenia gravis

*Consider **distribution** and whether **upper** or **lower motor neurone** or **muscular**.

GRADING POWER

Power, when tested, is graded conventionally using the Medical Research Council (MRC) scale. This is usually amended to divide grade 4 into 4+, 4 and 4−.

5	=normal power
4+	=submaximal movement against resistance
4	=moderate movement against resistance
4−	=slight movement against resistance
3	=moves against gravity but not resistance
2	=moves with gravity eliminated
1	=flicker
0	=no movement

Power should be graded according to the maximum power attained, no matter how briefly this is maintained.

WHAT TO DO

Look at the position of the patient overall.
- Look especially for a hemiplegic positioning, flexion of elbow and wrist with extension of knee and ankle.

Look for wasting.
- Compare the right side with the left side.

Look for fasciculation.
- Fasciculations are fine subcutaneous movements that represent contractions of a motor unit.

COMMON MISTAKES

- Fibrillations are spontaneous discharges from a single muscle fibre and are found on electromyography (EMG). They cannot be seen by the naked eye. Confusingly, fasciculations in the tongue have sometimes incorrectly been called fibrillations.

Test for tone.
Test muscle groups in a *systematic* way to test power.
Test reflexes.

Testing muscles of respiration and trunk muscles can be very important in specific situations. These are described in Chapter 25.

General comments

Always:

- Describe what to do in simple terms.
- Demonstrate the movements you require.
- Test simple movements across single joints.
- Fix or hold the joint to isolate the movement you want to test.
- Allow the patient to move the joint through the full range before testing power. When testing power, look at or feel the muscle contract.
- Compare the strength of the right side with the left side.
- Do not be afraid to repeat power tests so as to be certain of your findings.
- Think about what you are finding as you do the examination. It can be useful to 'summarise' what you find in your head as you do the examination. This makes it easier when you come to write your findings down in the notes (or report them to an examiner!).

MOTOR SYSTEM: 16

TONE

BACKGROUND

Testing muscle tone is a very important indicator of the presence and site of pathology. It can be surprisingly difficult to evaluate.

WHAT TO DO

Ensure the patient is relaxed, or at least distracted by conversation. Repeat each movement at different speeds.

Arms

Take the hand as if to shake it and hold the forearm. First pronate and supinate the forearm. Then roll the hand round at the wrist (Fig. 16.1). Hold the forearm and the elbow and move the arm through the full range of flexion and extension at the elbow.

Legs

Tone at the hip
The patient is lying with straight legs. Roll the knee from side to side (Fig. 16.2).

Tone at the knee
Put your hand behind the knee and lift it rapidly. Watch the heel. Hold the knee and ankle. Flex and extend the knee.

Tone at the ankle
Hold the ankle and flex and dorsiflex the foot.

COMMON MISTAKES

Patients fail to relax. This is usually worsened by commands to relax and improved by irrelevant conversations or asking the patient to count down from 100.

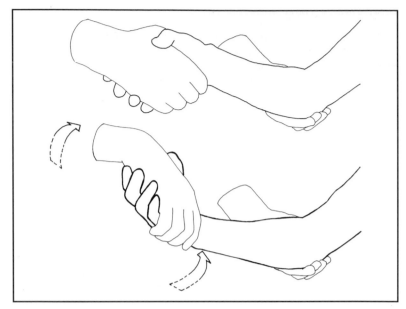

Figure 16.1
Roll the wrist

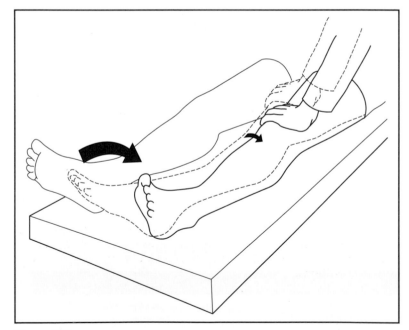

Figure 16.2
Roll the knee

WHAT YOU FIND

- *Normal*: slight resistance through whole range of movements. Heel will lift minimally off the bed.
- *Decreased tone*: loss of resistance through movement. Heel does not lift off the bed when the knee is lifted quickly. Marked loss of tone = flaccid.
- *Increased tone*:
  - Resistance increases suddenly ('the catch'); the heel easily leaves the bed when the knee is lifted quickly: *spasticity*.
  - Increased through whole range, as if bending a lead pipe: *lead pipe rigidity*. Regular intermittent break in tone through whole range: *cogwheel rigidity*.
  - Patient apparently opposes your attempts to move his limb: *Gegenhalten* or *paratonia*.

Special situations

- **Myotonia**: slow relaxation following action. Demonstrated by asking the patient to make a fist and then release it suddenly. In myotonia the hand will only unfold slowly.
- **Dystonia**: patient maintains posture at extreme of movement with contraction of agonist and antagonist (see Chapter 24).
- **Percussion myotonia**: may be demonstrated when a muscle dimples following percussion with a patella hammer. Most commonly sought in abductor pollicis brevis and the tongue.

WHAT IT MEANS

- **Flaccidity** or reduced tone. *Common causes*: lower motor neurone or cerebellar lesion. *Rare causes*: myopathies, 'spinal shock' (e.g. early after a stroke), chorea.
- **Spasticity**: upper motor lesion. This usually takes some time to develop.
- **Rigidity and cogwheel rigidity**: extrapyramidal syndromes. *Common causes*: Parkinson's disease, phenothiazines.
- **Gegenhalten** or **paratonia**: bilateral frontal lobe damage. *Common causes*: cerebrovascular disease, dementia.
- **Myotonia** (rare). *Causes*: myotonic dystrophy (associated with frontal balding, ptosis, cataracts and cardiac conduction defects) and myotonia congenita. Percussion myotonia may be found in both conditions.

MOTOR SYSTEM:

ARMS

17

BACKGROUND

Upper motor neurone or pyramidal weakness predominantly affects finger extension, elbow extension and shoulder abduction. N.B. Elbow flexion and grip are relatively preserved.

Muscles are usually innervated by more than one nerve root. The exact distribution varies between individuals. The main root innervations and reflexes are shown in simplified form in Table 17.1. More detailed root distribution is given below.

Table 17.1
Nerve roots: simplified root innervations and main reflexes

Root	Movements	Reflex
C5	Shoulder abduction, elbow flexion	Biceps
C6	Elbow flexion (semi-pronated)	Supinator
C7	Finger extension, elbow extension	Triceps
C8	Finger flexors	Finger
T1	Small muscles of the hand	No reflex

The three nerves of greatest clinical importance in the arm are the radial, ulnar and median nerves.

- The **radial nerve** and its branches supply all extensors in the arm.
- The **ulnar nerve** supplies all intrinsic hand muscles except 'LOAF' (see below).
- The **median nerve** supplies:
  - L lateral two lumbricals
  - O opponens pollicis
  - A abductor pollicis brevis
  - F flexor pollicis brevis.

N.B. All intrinsic hand muscles are supplied by T1.

WHAT TO DO

Look at the arms

Note wasting and fasciculations, especially in the shoulder girdle, deltoid and small muscles of the hands (the first dorsal interossei and abductor pollicis brevis).

Test tone (see Chapter 15).

PRONATOR TEST

Ask the patient to hold his arms out in front with his palms facing upwards and to close his eyes tightly (*demonstrate*).
   Watch the position of the arms.

What you find and what it means:
- One arm pronates and drifts downwards: indicates *weakness on that side.*
- Both arms drift downwards: indicates *bilateral weakness.*
- Arm rises: suggests *cerebellar disease.*
- Fingers   continuously   move   up   and   down— pseudoathetosis—indicates *deficit of joint position sense.*

Basic screening examination

A simple screening procedure is outlined below. Some further muscle power tests are given afterwards. Perform each test on one side, then compare to the other side.

Shoulder abduction
Ask the patient to lift both his elbows out to the side (*demonstrate*). Ask him to push up (Fig. 17.1).

- *Muscle*: deltoid
- *Nerve*: axillary nerve
- *Root*: C5.

Elbow flexion
Hold the patient's elbow and wrist. Ask him to pull his hand towards his face. N.B. Ensure the arm is supinated (Fig. 17.2).

- *Muscle*: biceps brachii
- *Nerve*: musculocutaneous nerve
- *Root*: C5, C6.

(Trick movement involves pronation of the arm to use brachioradialis— see below.)

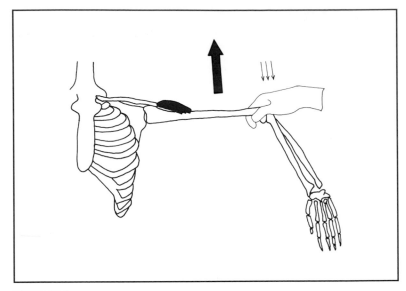

Figure 17.1
Testing shoulder abduction

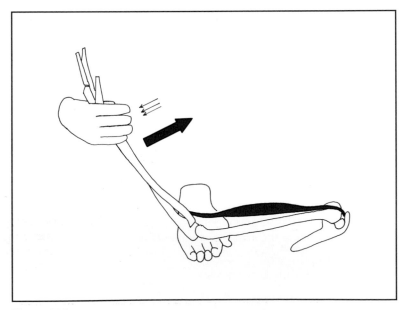

Figure 17.2
Testing elbow flexion

Elbow extension

Hold the patient's elbow and wrist. Ask him to extend the elbow (Fig. 17.3).

- *Muscle*: triceps
- *Nerve*: radial nerve
- *Root*: (C6), C7, (C8).

Wrist extension

Hold the patient's forearm. Ask him to make a fist and bend his wrist up (Fig. 17.4).

- *Muscle*: flexor carpi ulnaris and radialis
- *Nerve*: radial nerve
- *Root*: (C6), C7, (C8).

Finger extension

Fix the patient's hand. Ask him to keep his fingers straight. Press against the extended fingers (Fig. 17.5).

- *Muscle*: extensor digitorum
- *Nerve*: posterior interosseous nerve (a branch of the radial nerve)
- *Root*: C7, (C8).

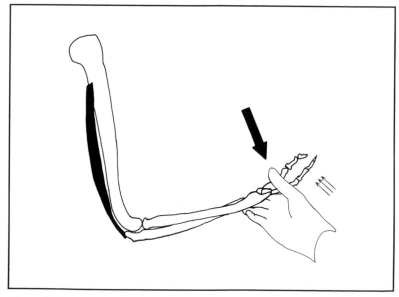

Figure 17.3
Testing elbow extension

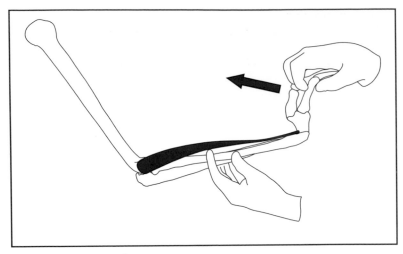

Figure 17.4
Testing wrist extension

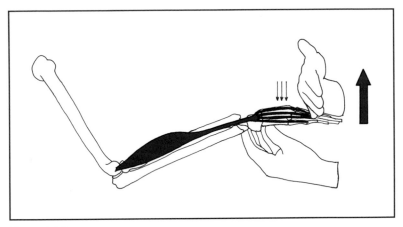

Figure 17.5
Testing finger extension

Finger flexion

Close your fingers on the patient's fingers palm to palm so that both sets of fingertips are on the other's metacarpal phalangeal joints. Ask the patient to grip your fingers and then attempt to open the patient's grip (Fig. 17.6).

- *Muscles*: flexor digitorum superficialis and profundus
- *Nerves*: median and ulnar nerves
- *Root*: C8.

Finger abduction

Ask the patient to spread his fingers out (*demonstrate*). Ensure the palm is in line with the fingers. Hold the middle of the little fingers and attempt to overcome the index finger (Fig. 17.7).

- *Muscle*: first dorsal interosseous
- *Nerve*: ulnar nerve
- *Root*: T1.

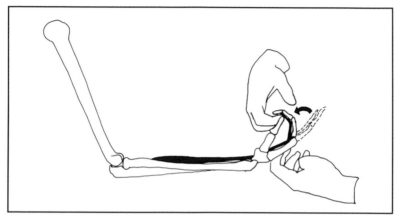

Figure 17.6
Testing finger flexion

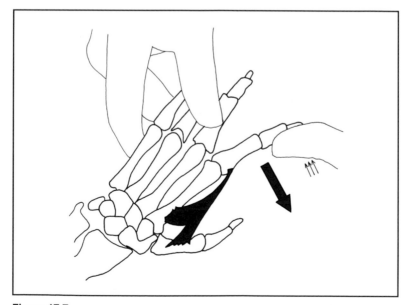

Figure 17.7
Testing finger abduction

Finger adduction

Ask the patient to bring his fingers together. Make sure the fingers are straight. Fix the middle, ring and little fingers. Attempt to abduct the index finger (Fig. 17.8).

- *Muscle*: second palmar interosseous
- *Nerve*: ulnar nerve
- *Root*: T1.

Thumb abduction

Ask the patient to place his palm flat with a supinated arm. Ask him then to bring his thumb towards his nose. Fix the palm and, pressing at the end of the proximal phalanx joint, attempt to overcome the resistance (Fig. 17.9).

- *Muscle*: abductor pollicis brevis
- *Nerve*: median
- *Root*: T1.

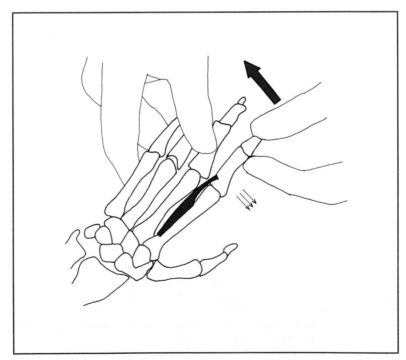

Figure 17.8
Testing finger adduction

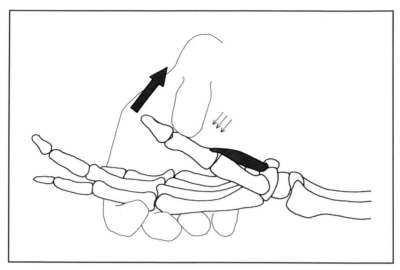

Figure 17.9
Testing thumb abduction

FURTHER TESTS OF ARM POWER

These tests are performed in the light of the clinical abnormality.

Serratus anterior
Stand behind the patient in front of a wall. Ask him to push against the wall with his arms straight and his hands at shoulder level. Look at the position of the scapula. If the muscle is weak, the scapula lifts off the chest wall: 'winging' (Fig. 17.10).

- *Nerve*: long thoracic nerve
- *Root*: C5, C6, C7.

Rhomboids
Ask the patient to put his hands on his hips. Hold his elbow and ask him to bring his elbow backwards (Fig. 17.11).

- *Muscle*: rhomboids
- *Nerve*: nerve to rhomboids
- *Root*: C4, C5.

Supraspinatus
Stand behind the patient. Ask the patient to lift his arm from the side against resistance (Fig. 17.12).

- *Nerve*: suprascapular nerve
- *Root*: C5.

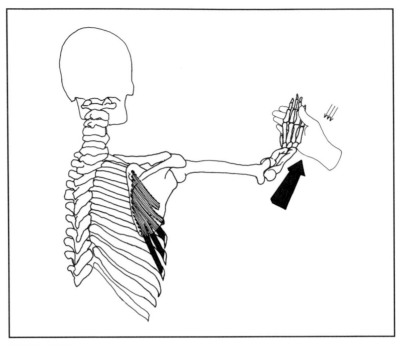

Figure 17.10
Testing strength of serratus anterior

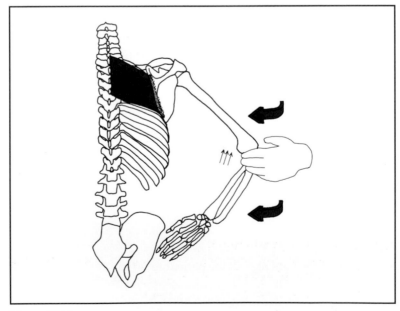

Figure 17.11
Testing strength of rhomboids

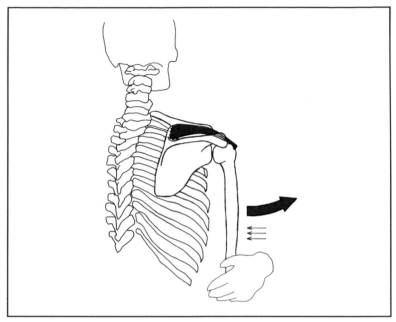

Figure 17.12
Testing strength of supraspinatus

Infraspinatus
Stand behind the patient, hold his elbow against his side with the elbow flexed, asking him to keep his elbow in and move his hand out to the side. Resist this with your hand at his wrist (Fig. 17.13).

- *Nerve*: suprascapular nerve
- *Root*: C5, C6.

Brachioradialis
Hold the patient's forearm and wrist with the forearm semi-pronated (as if shaking hands). Ask the patient to pull his hand towards his face (Fig. 17.14).

- *Muscle*: brachioradialis
- *Nerve*: radial nerve
- *Root*: C6.

Long flexors of little and ring finger
Ask the patient to grip your fingers. Attempt to extend the distal interphalangeal joint of the little and ring fingers.

- *Muscle*: flexor digitorum profundus 3 and 4
- *Nerve*: ulnar nerve
- *Root*: C8.

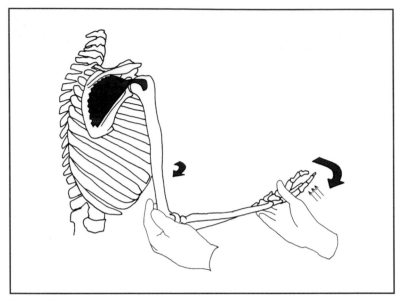

Figure 17.13
Testing strength of infraspinatus

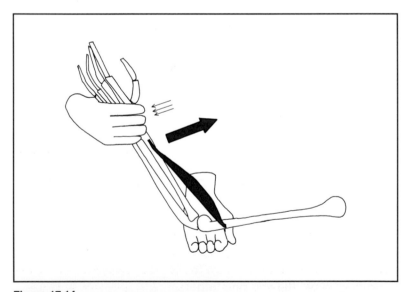

Figure 17.14
Testing strength of brachioradialis

WHAT YOU FIND

This will be considered in Chapter 20.

MOTOR SYSTEM:

18

LEGS

BACKGROUND

Upper motor neurone or pyramidal weakness predominantly affects hip flexion, knee flexion and foot dorsiflexion.

Simplified root distribution in the legs is shown in Table 18.1

Table 18.1
Simplified root distribution in the legs

Nerve roots	Movement	Reflex
L1, L2	Hip flexion	No reflex
L3, L4	Knee extension	Knee reflex
L5	Dorsiflexion of foot, inversion and eversion of ankle, extension of great toe	No reflex
S1	Hip extension, knee flexion, plantarflexion	Ankle reflex

Femoral nerve supplies knee extension.
Sciatic nerve supplies knee flexion. Its branches are:

- Posterior tibial branch—supplies foot plantarflexion and inversion and the small muscles of the foot.
- Common peroneal branch—supplies dorsiflexion and eversion of the ankle.

WHAT TO DO

Look at the legs for wasting and fasciculation.

Note especially the quadriceps, the anterior compartment of the shin, the extensor digitorum and brevis, and the peroneal muscles.

Look for the position and for contractures, especially at the ankle; **look at the shape of the foot**, a high arch or pes cavus.

Pes cavus is demonstrated by holding a hard, flat surface against the sole of the foot; a gap can be seen between the foot and the surface.

Power testing screening

Compare the left with the right.

Hip flexion

Ask the patient to lift his knee towards his chest. When the knee is at 90 degrees, ask him to pull it up as hard as he can; put your hand against his knee and try to overcome this (Fig. 18.1).

- *Muscle*: iliopsoas
- *Nerve*: lumbar sacral plexus
- *Root*: L1, L2.

Hip extension

The patient is lying flat with his legs straight. Put your hand under his heel and ask him to push down to press your hand (Fig. 18.2).

- *Muscle*: gluteus maximus
- *Nerve*: inferior gluteal nerve
- *Root*: L5, S1.

Knee extension

Ask the patient to bend his knee. When it is flexed at 90 degrees, support the knee with one hand and place the other hand at his ankle and ask him to straighten his leg (Fig. 18.3).

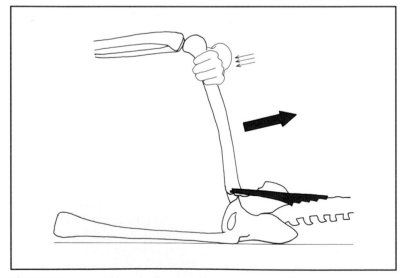

Figure 18.1
Testing hip flexion

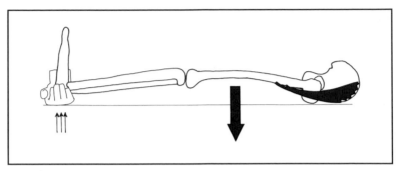

Figure 18.2
Testing hip extension

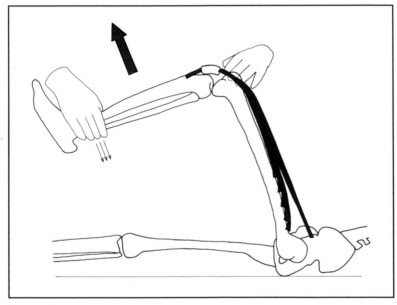

Figure 18.3
Testing knee extension

- *Muscle*: quadriceps femoris
- *Nerve*: femoral nerve
- *Root*: L3, L4.

Knee flexion

Ask the patient to bend his knee and bring his heel towards his bottom. When the knee is at 90 degrees, try to straighten the leg while holding the knee. Watch the hamstring muscles (Fig. 18.4).

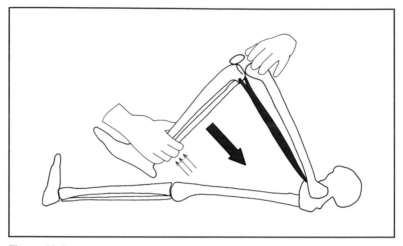

Figure 18.4
Testing knee flexion

- *Muscles*: hamstrings
- *Nerve*: sciatic nerve
- *Root*: L5, S1.

Foot dorsiflexion
Ask the patient to cock his ankle back and bring his toes towards his head. When the ankle is past 90 degrees, try to overcome this movement. Watch the anterior compartment of the leg (Fig. 18.5).

- *Muscle*: tibialis anterior
- *Nerve*: deep peroneal nerve
- *Root*: L4, L5.

Plantar flexion of the foot
Ask the patient to point his toes with his leg straight. Try to overcome this (Fig. 18.6).

- *Muscle*: gastrocnemius
- *Nerve*: posterior tibial nerve
- *Root*: S1.

Big toe extension
Ask the patient to pull his big toe up towards his face. Try to push the distal phalanx of his big toe down (Fig. 18.7).

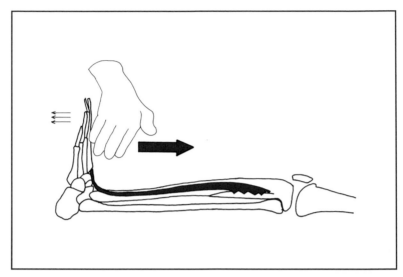

Figure 18.5
Testing dorsiflexion of the foot

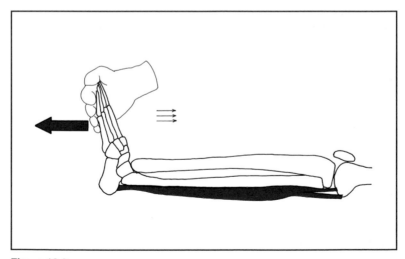

Figure 18.6
Testing plantar flexion of the foot

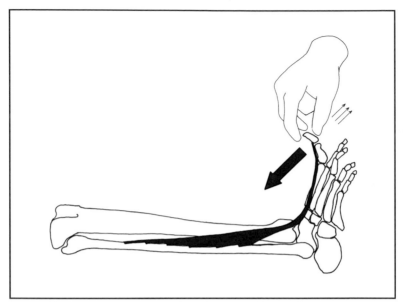

Figure 18.7
Testing big toe extension

- *Muscle*: extensor hallucis longus
- *Nerve*: deep peroneal nerve
- *Root*: L5.

Extension of the toes
Ask the patient to bring all his toes towards his head. Press against the proximal part of his toes; watch the muscle (Fig. 18.8).

- *Muscle*: extensor digitorum brevis
- *Nerve*: deep peroneal nerve
- *Root*: L5, S1.

Additional tests
Hip abductors
Fix one ankle; ask the patient to push the other leg out at the side and resist this movement by holding the other ankle (Fig. 18.9).

- *Muscle*: gluteus medius and minimus
- *Nerve*: superior gluteal nerve
- *Root*: L4, L5.

Hip adductors
Ask the patient to keep his ankles together. Fix one ankle and try to pull the other ankle out (Fig. 18.10).

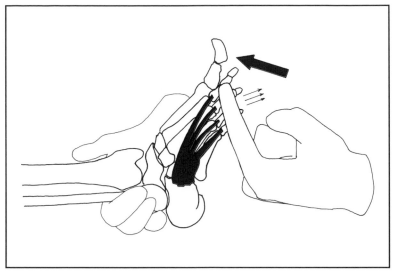

Figure 18.8
Testing extension of the toes

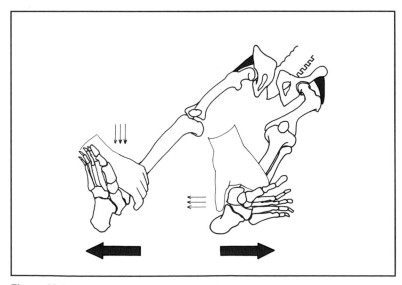

Figure 18.9
Testing strength of hip abductors

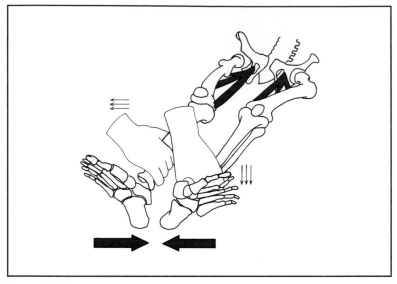

Figure 18.10
Testing strength of right hip adductors

- *Muscle*: adductors
- *Nerve*: obturator nerve
- *Root*: L2, L3.

Foot inversion

With the ankle at 90 degrees, ask the patient to turn his foot inwards. This frequently requires demonstration (Fig. 18.11).

- *Muscle*: tibialis posterior
- *Nerve*: tibial nerve
- *Root*: L4, L5.

Foot eversion

Ask the patient to turn his foot out to the side. Then try to bring the foot to the midline (Fig. 18.12).

- *Muscle*: peroneus longus and brevis
- *Nerve*: superficial peroneal nerve
- *Root*: L5, S1.

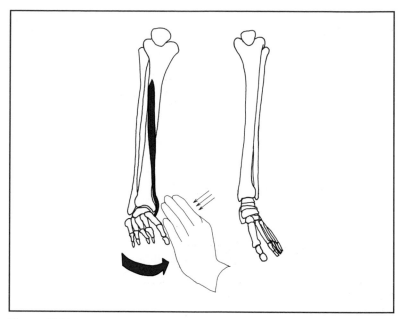

Figure 18.11
Testing inversion of the foot

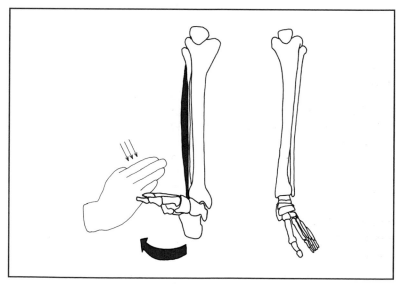

Figure 18.12
Testing eversion of the foot

REFLEXES

BACKGROUND

A tendon reflex results from the stimulation of a stretch-sensitive afferent from a neuromuscular spindle which, via a single synapse, stimulates a motor nerve, leading to a muscle contraction. Tendon reflexes are increased in upper motor neurone lesions and decreased in lower motor neurone lesions and muscle abnormalities.

The root values for the reflexes can be recalled by counting from the ankle upwards (Fig. 19.1).

Reflexes can be graded:

```
0   = absent
±   = present only with reinforcement
1+  = present but depressed
2+  = normal
3+  = increased
4+  = clonus.
```

WHAT TO DO

Use the whole length of the patella hammer; let the hammer swing. Ensure the patient is relaxed. Avoid telling the patient to relax, as this is guaranteed to produce tension.

Biceps
Place the patient's hands on his abdomen. Place your index finger on the biceps tendon; swing the hammer on to your finger while watching the biceps muscle (Fig. 19.2).

- *Nerve*: musculocutaneous nerve
- *Root*: C5, (C6).

Supinator
(N.B. Bad name for this reflex; the muscle involved is brachioradialis.)

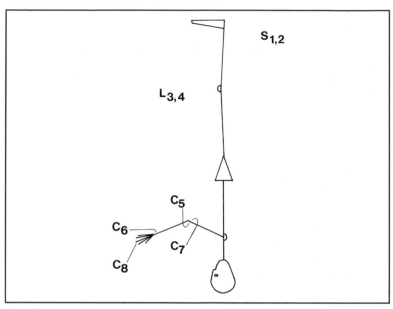

Figure 19.1
Reflex man. Simple as counting—start from the feet

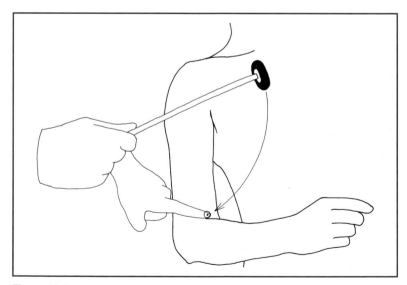

Figure 19.2
Testing the biceps reflex

Place the arm flexed on to the abdomen, place the finger on the radial tuberosity, hit the finger with the hammer and watch the brachioradialis (Fig. 19.3).

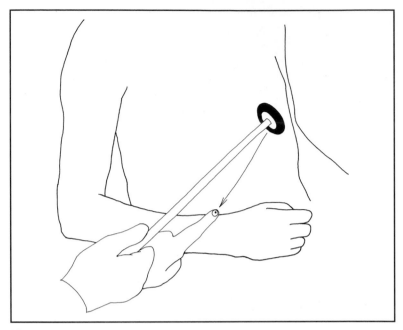

Figure 19.3
Testing the supinator reflex

- *Nerve*: radial nerve
- *Root*: C6, (C5).

Triceps

Draw the arm across the chest, holding the wrist with the elbow at 90 degrees. Strike the triceps tendon directly with the patella hammer; watch the muscle (Fig. 19.4).

- *Nerve*: radial nerve
- *Root*: C7.

Finger reflex

Hold the hand in the neutral position, place your hand opposite the fingers and strike the back of your fingers.

- *Muscle*: flexor digitorum profundus and superficialis
- *Nerve*: median and ulnar
- *Root*: C8.

Knee reflex

Place the arm under the knee so that the knee is at 90 degrees. Strike the knee below the patella; watch the quadriceps (Fig. 19.5).

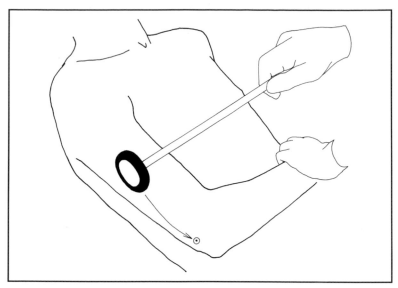

Figure 19.4
Testing the triceps reflex

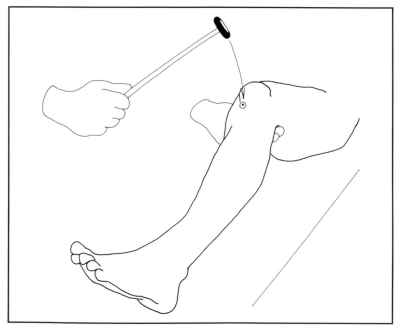

Figure 19.5
Testing the knee reflex

- *Nerve*: femoral nerve
- *Root*: L3–L4.

Ankle reflex

Hold the patient's foot at 90 degrees with a medial malleolus facing the ceiling. The knee should be flexed and lying to the side. Strike the Achilles tendon directly. Watch the muscles of the calf (Fig. 19.6A).

- *Nerve*: tibial nerve
- *Root*: S1–S2.

Ankle reflex alternatives

1. With the patient's legs straight, place your hand on the ball of his foot with the ankles at 90 degrees. Strike with your hand and watch the muscles of the calf (Fig. 19.6B).
2. Ask the patient to kneel on a chair so that his ankles are hanging loose over the edge. Strike the Achilles tendon directly (Fig. 19.6C).

Reinforcement

If any reflex is unobtainable directly, ask the patient to perform a reinforcement manœuvre. For the arms, ask the patient to clench his teeth as you swing the hammer. For the legs, ask the patient either to make a fist, or to link hands across his chest and pull one against the other, as you swing the hammer (Fig. 19.7).

COMMON MISTAKES

- Patient will not relax. Ask diverting questions: where he comes from, how long he has lived there, and so on.
- Tendon hammer not swung but stabbed: hold the hammer correctly.

 TIP   An absent reflex sounds dull. It's worth listening as well as watching.

Further manœuvres

Demonstration of clonus

- **At the ankle**: Dorsiflex the ankle briskly; maintain the foot in that position and a rhythmic contraction may be found. More than three beats is abnormal.
- **At the knee**: With the leg straight, take the patella and bring it briskly downwards; a rhythmic contraction may be noted. Always abnormal.

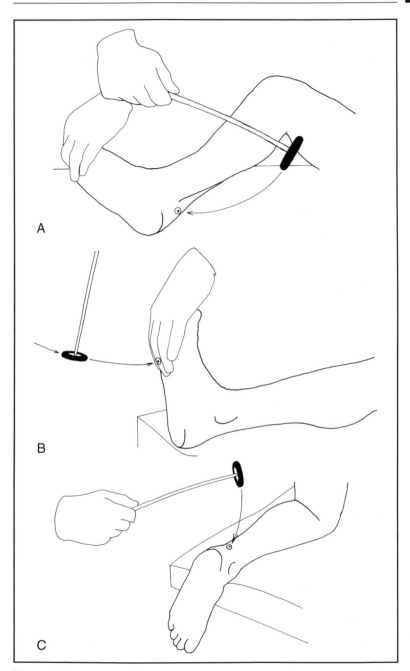

Figure 19.6
The ankle reflex—three ways to get it

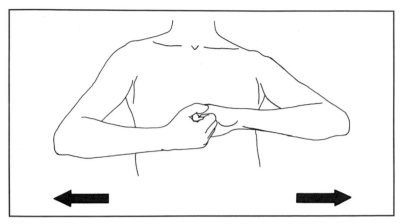

Figure 19.7
Reinforcement

WHAT YOU FIND AND WHAT IT MEANS

- **Increased reflex or clonus**: this indicates an upper motor neurone lesion above the root at that level.
- Absent reflexes:
  - *generalised*: indicates peripheral neuropathy
  - *isolated*: indicates either a peripheral nerve or, more commonly, a root lesion
  - *bilateral absent ankle reflexes*: most commonly indicates a peripheral neuropathy; also occurs with bilateral S1 nerve root lesions or, very rarely, bilateral sciatic nerve lesions.
- **Reduced reflexes** (more difficult to judge): occurs in a peripheral neuropathy, muscle disease and cerebellar syndrome. N.B. Reflexes can be absent in the early stages of severe upper motor neurone lesion: 'spinal shock'.
- **Reflex spread**: the reflex tested is present but this response goes beyond the muscle normally seen to contract; for example, the fingers are seen to flex when the supinator reflex is tested or the hip adductors are seen to contract when testing the knee reflex. Reflex spread indicates an upper motor neurone lesion occurring above the level of innervation of the muscle to which the reflex spread.
- **An inverted reflex**: a combination of loss of the reflex tested with reflex spread to muscle at a lower level. The level of the absent reflex indicates the level of the lesion. For example, a biceps reflex is absent but produces a triceps response. This indicates a lower motor neurone lesion at the level of the absent reflex (in this case C5) with an upper motor neurone lesion below indicating spinal cord involvement at the level of the absent reflex.

- **Pendular reflex**: this is usually best seen in the knee jerk where the reflex continues to swing for several beats. This is associated with cerebellar disease.
- **Slow relaxing reflex**: this is especially seen at the ankle reflex and may be difficult to note. It is associated with hypothyroidism.

ABDOMINAL REFLEXES

What to do
Using an orange stick, lightly scratch the abdominal wall as indicated in Figure 19.8. Watch the abdominal wall; this should contract on the same side.

- *Afferents*: segmental sensory nerves
- *Efferents*: segmental motor nerves
- *Roots*: above the umbilicus, T8–T9; below the umbilicus, T10–T11.

What you find and what it means
- **Abdominal reflex absent**: obesity, previous abdominal operations or frequent pregnancy, age, a pyramidal tract involvement above that level or a peripheral nerve abnormality.

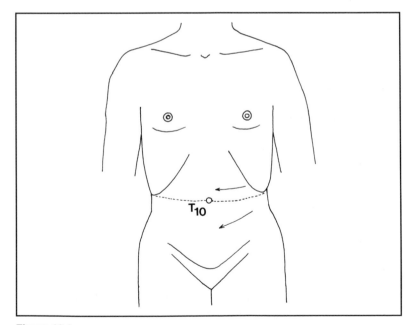

Figure 19.8
Abdominal reflexes

PLANTAR RESPONSE

What to do

Explain to the patient that you are going to stroke the bottom part of his foot. Gently draw an orange stick up a lateral border of the foot and across the foot pad. Watch the big toe and the remainder of the foot (Fig. 19.9).

What you find

- The toes all flex—flexor plantar response: *negative Babinski's sign—normal.*
- Hallux extends (goes up), the other toes flex or spread: extensor plantar response or *positive Babinski's sign.*
- Hallux extends (goes up), the other toes extend and ankle dorsiflexes: *withdrawal response.* Repeat more gently or try alternative stimuli (see below).
- No movement of the hallux (even if the other toes flex): indicates *no response.*
- A positive test should be reproducible.

What it means

- **Extensor plantar response**: indicates upper motor neurone lesion.
- **Flexor plantar response**: normal.

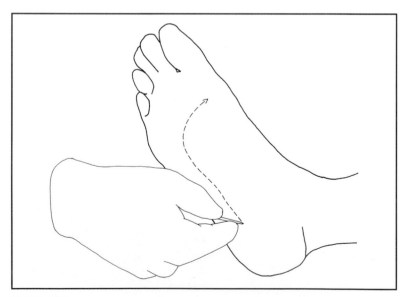

Figure 19.9
Testing the plantar response

- **No response**: may occur with profound upper motor neurone weakness (toe unable to extend); may occur if there is a sensory abnormality interfering with the afferent part of the reflex.

COMMON MISTAKES

Do not place too much weight on the plantar response in isolation. A flexor plantar response may be found in an upper motor neurone lesion. An extensor plantar response which surprises you (one that doesn't fit the rest of the clinical picture) needs to be interpreted with caution—could it be a withdrawal response?

Alternative stimuli (all trying to elicit the same responses)
- Stimulus on lateral aspect of foot: *Chaddock's reflex*.
- Thumb and index finger run down the medial aspect of the tibia: *Oppenheim's reflex*.

These alternative stimuli are only useful *if present,* not if absent.

MOTOR SYSTEM:

20

WHAT YOU FIND AND WHAT IT MEANS

WHAT YOU FIND

Remember:

- **Upper motor neurone pattern**: increased tone, brisk reflexes, pyramidal pattern of weakness, extensor plantar responses.
- **Lower motor neurone pattern**: wasting, fasciculation, decreased tone, decreased or absent reflexes, flexor plantar responses.
- **Muscle disease**: wasting (usually proximal), decreased tone, decreased or absent reflexes, flexor plantars.
- **Neuromuscular junction**: fatigable weakness, normal or decreased tone, normal reflexes, flexor plantars.
- **Functional weakness**: no wasting, normal tone, normal reflexes, flexor plantars, erratic power.

See Figure 20.1.

> ✔ **TIP**   Making full sense of the motor signs will also depend on sensory and other signs.

1. Weakness in all four limbs
a. With increased reflexes and extensor plantar responses
- Anatomical localisation: cervical cord lesion or bilateral pyramidal lesions.

> ✔ **TIP**   Sensory testing and cranial nerve signs may be used to discriminate.

b. With absent reflexes
- Polyradiculopathy, peripheral neuropathy or a myopathy. Sensory testing should be normal in a myopathy.

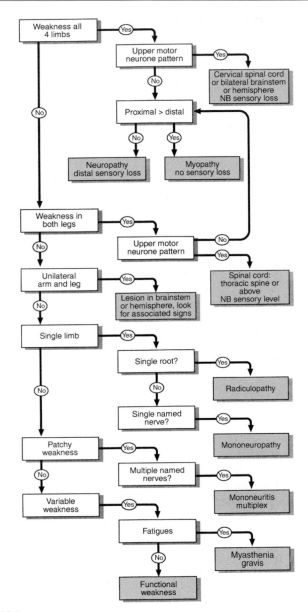

Figure 20.1
Flow chart: simplified approach to weakness

> **TIP**   In the state of 'spinal shock' that occurs after a recent acute and severe upper motor neurone lesion, tone will be reduced and reflexes may be absent—even though this in an upper motor neurone lesion.

c. Mixed upper motor neurone (in the legs) and lower motor neurone weakness (in the arms)
- Suggests motor neurone disease (which has no sensory loss) or mixed cervical myelopathy and radiculopathy (with sensory loss).

d. Normal reflexes
- Fatigable weakness, particularly with associated cranial nerve abnormalities (eye movements, ptosis, facial muscles): *myasthenia gravis.*
- Variable weakness, normal tone: consider *functional non-organic weakness.*

2. Weakness in both legs
a. With increased reflexes and extensor plantar responses
- Suggests a lesion in the spinal cord. The lesion must be above the root level of the highest motor abnormality. A level may be ascertained with sensory signs.

b. With absent reflexes in the legs
- Polyradiculopathy, cauda equina lesions or peripheral neuropathy.

3. Unilateral arm and leg weakness
Upper motor neurone lesion in the high cervical cord, brainstem or above
- Contralateral sensory findings (pain and temperature loss) indicate lesion of half ipsilateral cervical cord lesion (Brown–Séquard) (see Chapter 21).
- Contralateral cranial nerve lesions or brainstem signs indicate the level of brainstem affected.
- Ipsilateral facial or tongue weakness indicate lesion above brainstem.
- Ipsilateral sensory loss indicate a lesion above the medulla.
- Visual field or higher function deficits indicate hemisphere lesion.

> **TIP**   Associated cranial nerve, visual field defect or higher function defect may allow more accurate localisation.

4. Syndromes limited to a single limb
Upper motor neurone signs limited to a single limb can be caused by lesions in the spinal cord, brainstem or cerebral hemisphere. Motor signs alone cannot distinguish between these possibilities. This relies on other signs—for example, cranial nerve or sensory abnormalities— or a diagnosis may not be possible without further investigation.

If lower motor neurone, common syndromes seen are as follows.

a. Upper limb
Hand
(i) *Median nerve*: weakness and wasting of thenar eminence abductor pollicis brevis. *Sensory loss*: thumb, index and middle finger (Chapter 21).
(ii) *Ulnar nerve*: weakness with or without wasting of all muscles in hand excepting the LOAF. *Sensory loss*: little and half ring finger (Chapter 21).
(iii) *T1 root*: wasting of all small muscles of the hand. N.B. Sensory changes are confined to the medial forearm.
(iv) *Radial nerve*: weakness of finger extension, wrist extension and probably triceps and brachioradialis. *Minimal sensory changes* at anatomical snuffbox. *Reflex loss*: supinator; triceps may also be lost if lesion above spiral groove.
(v) Bilateral wasting of small muscles:
  – *with distal sensory loss*: peripheral neuropathy
  – *without sensory loss*: motor neurone disease.

Arm
(i) *C5 root*: weakness of shoulder abduction, external rotation and elbow flexion; loss of biceps reflex. *Sensory loss*: outer aspect of upper arm (Chapter 21).
(ii) *C6 root*: weakness of elbow flexion, pronation; loss of supinator reflex. *Sensory loss*: lateral aspect of forearm and thumb (Chapter 21).
(iii) *C7 root*: weakness of elbow and wrist extension; loss of triceps reflex. *Sensory loss*: middle finger (Chapter 21). N.B. cf. radial nerve.
(iv) *C8 root*: weakness of finger flexion; loss of finger reflex. *Sensory loss*: medial aspect of forearm (Chapter 21).
(v) *Axillary nerve*: weakness of shoulder abduction (deltoid). *Sensory loss*: small patch on lateral part of shoulder (Chapter 21).

b. Lower limb
(i) *Common peroneal palsy*: weakness of foot dorsiflexion and eversion with preserved inversion. *Sensory loss*: lateral shin and dorsum of foot (Chapter 21). N.B. cf. L5 root.
(ii) *L4 root*: weakness of knee extension and foot dorsiflexion. *Reflex loss*: knee reflex. *Sensory loss*: medial shin (Chapter 21).

(iii) *L5 root*: weakness of foot dorsiflexion, inversion and eversion, extension of the big toe and hip abduction. *Sensory loss*: lateral shin and dorsum of foot (Chapter 21).

(iv) *S1 root*: weakness of plantar flexion, and foot eversion. *Reflex loss*: ankle reflex. *Sensory loss*: lateral border of foot, sole of foot (Chapter 21).

5. Variable weakness

 (i) Weakness seems to fatigue with effort then recovers: consider myasthenia gravis.

(ii) Fluctuates, with effort collapsing at times and at other times giving full power: consider functional weakness.

6. Weakness that is not really there

Patients may appear weak when they are not, if:

- They find it difficult to understand what you want them to do (altered higher function).
- They are slow to initiate movements (bradykinesia as in Parkinson's disease).
- The movement is painful.
- They are not sure where their limb is due to proprioceptive loss.

If in doubt, re-examine them with these factors in mind.

WHAT IT MEANS

Myopathy (rare)

Causes

- **Inherited**: muscular dystrophies (Duchenne's, Becker's, fascio-scapular-humeral, myotonic dystrophy).
- **Inflammatory**: polymyositis, dermatomyositis, polymyalgia rheumatica.
- **Endocrine**: steroid-induced, hyperthyroid, hypothyroid.
- **Metabolic**: (very rare) glycogen storage disease (e.g. Pompe's disease), McArdle's disease.
- **Toxic**: alcohol, statins, chloroquine, clofibrate.

Myasthenic syndromes (rare)

Causes

- **Myasthenia gravis**: usually idiopathic; occasionally drug-induced (penicillamine, hydralazine).
- **Lambert–Eaton syndrome:** (very rare) paraneoplastic syndrome (usually oat cell carcinoma).

Mononeuropathies (very common)

Common causes

- **Compression** (Saturday night palsy: compressing radial nerve in spiral groove by leaning arm over chair—also reported to affect sciatic nerve after falling asleep sitting on toilet!).
- **Entrapment**, e.g. median nerve in carpel tunnel, common peroneal nerve behind head of fibula at the knee; more common in diabetes mellitus, rheumatoid arthritis, hypothyroidism and acromegaly.
- May be presentation of more diffuse neuropathy.

Radiculopathies (common)

Common causes

- Cervical or lumbar disc protrusion. N.B. The root compressed is from the lower of the levels; for example, an L5/S1 disc compresses the S1 root. N.B. A radiculopathy may occur at the level of a compressive spinal lesion.

Rare causes

- Secondary tumours, neurofibromas.

Peripheral neuropathies (common)

- **Acute predominantly motor neuropathies**: Guillain–Barré syndrome. *Very rarely*: diphtheria, porphyria.
- **Subacute sensorimotor neuropathies**: vitamin deficiencies (B_1, B_{12}); heavy metal toxicity (lead, arsenic, thallium); drugs (vincristine, isoniazid); uraemia.
- Chronic sensorimotor neuropathies:
  - *Acquired*: diabetes mellitus; hypothyroidism; paraproteinaemias; amyloidosis.
  - *Inherited*: hereditary motor and sensory neuropathy (Charcot–Marie–Tooth disease).

Mononeuritis multiplex (rare)

- *Inflammatory*: polyarteritis nodosa, rheumatoid arthritis, systemic lupus erythematosus, sarcoidosis. N.B. May be presentation of more diffuse process.

Polyradiculopathy (rare)

Indicates lesion to many roots. It is distinct from other peripheral neuropathies because it produces a more proximal weakness. The term is commonly applied to Guillain–Barré syndrome.

Spinal cord syndromes (common)

Sensory findings are needed to interpret the significance of motor signs indicating a spinal cord syndrome (see Chapter 21).

Brainstem lesions (common)

- **Young patients.** *Common cause*: multiple sclerosis.
- **Older patients.** *Common causes*: brainstem infarction following emboli or thrombosis; haemorrhage. *Rarer causes*: tumours, trauma.

Hemisphere lesions (common)

- **Older patients.** *Common causes*: infarction following emboli or thrombosis; haemorrhage. *Rarer causes*: tumours, trauma, multiple sclerosis.

Functional weakness

Difficult to assess. May be an elaboration of an underlying organic weakness. May indicate conversion disorder or other somatoform disorders; cf. functional sensory loss.

SENSATION: 21

GENERAL

BACKGROUND

There are five basic modalities of sensation (Table 21.1).

Table 21.1
Modalities of sensation

Modality	Tract	Fibre size
Vibration sense Joint position sense Light touch	Posterior column	Large fibre
Pinprick Temperature	Spinothalamic tract	Small fibre

The posterior column remains ipsilateral up to the medulla, where it crosses over. The spinothalamic tract mostly crosses within one to two segments of entry (Fig. 21.1).

Vibration, joint position and temperature senses are often lost without prominent symptoms.

Light touch and pinprick loss is usually symptomatic.

Sensory examination should be used:

- as a screening test
- to assess the symptomatic patient
- to test hypotheses generated by motor examination (e.g. to distinguish between combined ulnar and median nerve lesions and a T1 root lesion).

Sensory examination requires considerable concentration on the part of both patient and examiner. Vibration sense and joint position sense are usually quick and easy and require little concentration, so test these first. This also allows you to assess the reliability of the patient as a sensory witness.

In all parts of sensory testing it is essential first to **teach** the patient about the test. Then perform the **test.** In most patients you will be confident they have understood and that their responses are reliable.

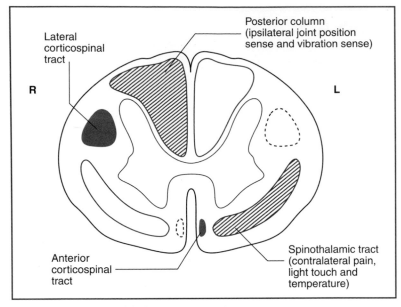

Figure 21.1
Spinal cord section showing sensory input (blue) from and motor output (black) to the right (R) side

Sometimes you will need to **check** that the patient has understood and carried out the test appropriately. With all testing, move from areas of sensory loss to areas of normal sensation.

Remember that sensory signs are 'softer' than reflex or motor changes; therefore less weight is generally given to them in synthesising these findings with associated motor and reflex changes.

Arms

There are four individual nerves which are commonly affected in the arm. The relevant sensory loss is illustrated in the fingers for the median nerve, ulnar nerve, radial nerve and axillary nerve (Fig. 21.2A–C). There may be loss beyond the core sensory distributions illustrated.

The dermatomal representation in the arms can be remembered easily if you recall that the middle finger of the hand is supplied by C7. This is illustrated in Figure 21.3.

Legs

Individual sensory deficit is most commonly seen in the following individual nerves:

- lateral cutaneous nerve of the thigh (Fig. 21.4A)
- common peroneal nerve (also referred to as the lateral popliteal nerve) (Fig. 21.4B)

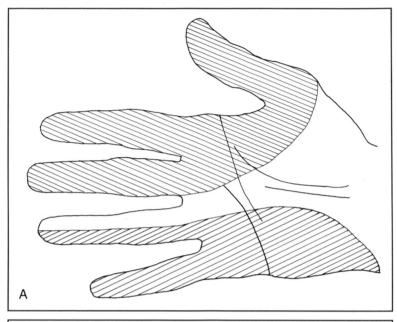

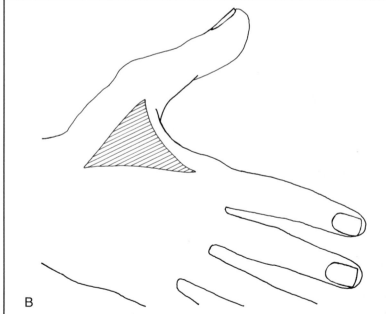

Figure 21.2
A. Sensory loss in the hand: median (blue) and ulnar (black) nerves
B. Sensory loss in the hand: radial nerve

(Continued)

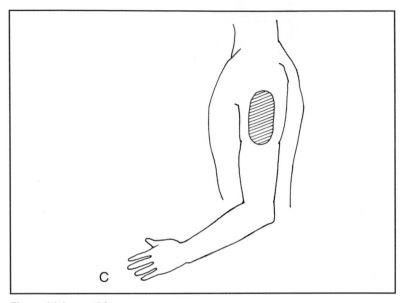

Figure 21.2, cont'd
C. Sensory loss in the arm: axillary nerve

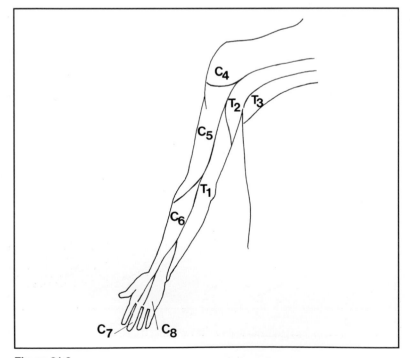

Figure 21.3
Dermatomes in the arm

- femoral nerve (Fig. 21.4C)
- sciatic nerve (Fig. 21.4D).

The dermatomes most frequently affected are L4, L5 and S1.

A 'dance' to help you remember the leg dermatomes is given in Figure 21.5.

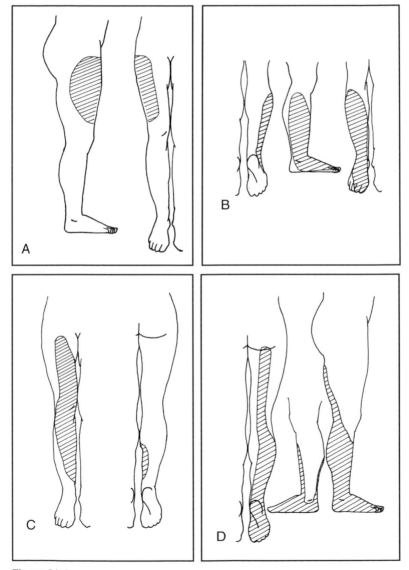

Figure 21.4
Sensory loss in the leg: **A.** Lateral cutaneous nerve of the thigh; **B.** Common peroneal nerve; **C.** Femoral nerve; **D.** Sciatic nerve

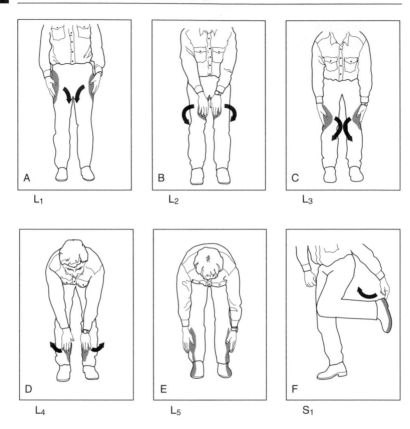

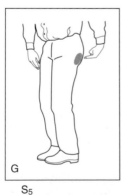

Figure 21.5
How to do the dermatomal dance: start with your hands over your pockets (L1), bring your hands IN to your inner thigh (L2), then OUT and down beside your knee (L3), then IN and down to your inner calf (L4), then OUT to your outer calf (L5) then point at the sole of your foot (S1), and point at your bottom (S5)

Dermatomes

An overview of the root innervation is given in Figure 21.6. The key dermatomes to be remembered are shown in blue.

WHAT TO DO

Vibration sense

Use a 128 Hz tuning fork. Those of higher frequency (256 or 512 Hz) are not adequate.

Demonstrate: ensure the patient understands that he is to feel a vibration, by striking the tuning fork and placing it on the sternum or chin.

Test: ask the patient to close his eyes. Place the tuning fork on the bony prominence and ask if he can feel the vibration. Place initially on the toe tips then, if this is not felt, on a metatarsal phalangeal joint, medial malleolus, tibial tuberosity, anterior superior iliac spine, in the arms, on the fingertips, each interphalangeal joint, the metacarpal phalangeal joint, the wrist, the elbow and the shoulder (Fig. 21.7). If sensation is normal distally, there is no point in proceeding proximally.

Check: check the patient reports feeling the vibration and not just the contact of the tuning fork. Strike the tuning fork and stop it vibrating immediately and repeat the test. If the patient reports that he feels vibration, demonstrate the test again.

N.B. Start distally and compare right with left.

Joint position sense

Demonstrate: with the patient's eyes open, show him what you are going to do. Hold the distal phalanx between your two fingers (Fig. 21.8). Ensuring that your fingers are at 90 degrees to the intended direction of movement, move the digit, illustrating which is up and which is down.

Test and check: ask the patient to close his eyes; move the toe up and down. Start with large movements in either direction; gradually reduce the angle moved until errors are made. Test distal joints first. Test more proximal joints if proprioception is abnormal distally, moving to more proximal joints until joint position sense is appreciated.

• *In the arm*: distal proximal interphalangeal joint, middle proximal interphalangeal joint, metacarpal phalangeal joint, wrist, elbow, shoulder.

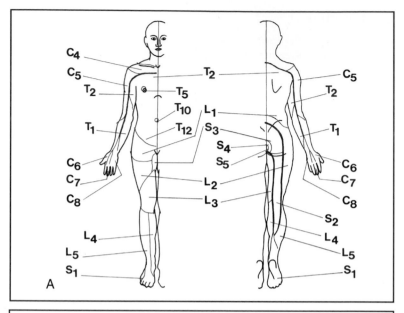

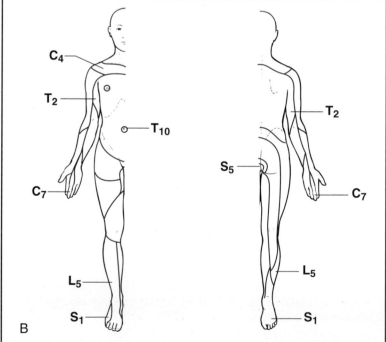

Figure 21.6
A. Overview of the dermatomes
B. Key dermatomes to remember

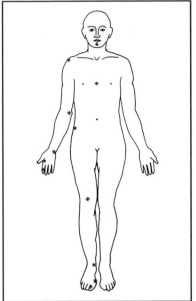

Figure 21.7
Potential sites for testing vibration sense

Figure 21.8
How to test joint position sense

 TIP   The size of movement normally detected is barely visible.

- *In the leg*: distal interphalangeal joint, metacarpal phalangeal joint, ankle, knee and hip.

 TIP   Romberg's test is a test for joint position sense (see Chapter 4).

COMMON MISTAKES

Make sure you hold the finger or toe by the sides (as in Fig. 21.8) and **not** the nail and pulp; otherwise you will test pressure appreciation as well as joint position sense.

Pinprick

Use a pin—a disposable neurological pin, or dressmaker's or safety pin—not a hypodermic needle or a broken orange stick. Dispose of the pin safely after use.

Try to produce a stimulus of the same intensity each time.

Demonstrate: show the patient what you are going to do. Explain that you want him to tell you if the pin is sharp or blunt. Touch an unaffected area with the pin and then touch an unaffected area with the opposite blunt end of the pin.

Test: ask the patient to close his eyes, then apply randomly sharp and blunt stimuli and note the patient's response.

Screening test
- Start distally and move proximally. Aim to stimulate points within each dermatome and each main nerve, though as a screening test this has a low yield.

Assessing a lesion
- Always start from the area of altered sensation and move towards normal to find the edges. Ask the patient to show you the area of abnormal sensation.

Assessing a hypothesis
- Test within the areas of interest with great care, particularly noting any difference between the two sides.

Check: intermittent use of a blunt stimulus that needs to be recognised correctly allows you to check that the patient understands the test.

 TIP   While you are testing pinprick, imagine how you would draw a picture of what you are finding for the patient's notes (as in Fig. 22.2).

Light touch

Use a piece of cotton wool. Some people prefer to use a fingertip. Dab this on to the skin. Try to ensure a repeatable stimulus. Avoid dragging it across the skin or tickling the patient.

Demonstrate: with the patient's eyes open, show him that you will be touching an area of skin. Ask him to say 'yes' every time he is touched.

Test: ask the patient to close his eyes; test the areas as for pinprick. Apply the stimulus at random intervals.

Check: Note the timing of the response to the irregular stimuli. Frequently a pause of 10–20 seconds may be useful.

Special situations

Sacral sensation: this is not usually screened. However, it is essential to test sacral sensation in any patient with:

• urinary or bowel symptoms
• bilateral leg weakness
• sensory loss in both legs
• a possible cord conus medullaris or cauda equina lesion.

Temperature sensation

Screening
It is usually adequate to ask a patient if the tuning fork feels cold when applied to the feet and hands. If cold is not appreciated, move the tuning fork proximally until it does feel cold.

Formal testing
Fill two tubes with warm water and cold water. Ideally these are controlled temperatures, though normally the warm and cold taps are adequate. Dry both tubes.
    Demonstrate: 'I want you to tell me if I touch you with the hot tube' (touch area of unaffected skin with the hot tube) 'or with the cold tube' (touch an unaffected area of skin with the cold tube).
    Test: Apply hot or cold at random to hands, feet or an affected area of interest.
    Check: the random order allows assessment of concentration.

COMMON MISTAKES

• **Generally**: Starting testing proximally rather than distally
• **Vibration sense and joint position sense**: Inadequate explanation, hurried testing without checking
• **Pinprick**: Drawing blood because of a non-blunted needle, varied pressure, calloused skin
• **Light touch**: Calloused skin, varied pressure
• **Pinprick and cotton wool**: Normal variations in sensory threshold may be interpreted as an abnormality

---

  TIP The ankle, knee, groin and axilla are all areas of relatively heightened sensitivity.

Other modalities

Two-point discrimination
This requires a two-point discriminator: a device like a blunted pair of compasses.

Demonstrate: 'I'm going to touch you with either two points together' (touch an unaffected area with the prongs set widely apart while the patient watches) 'or one point' (touch with one point). 'Now close your eyes.'

Test: gradually reduce the distance between the prongs, touching either with one or two prongs. Note the setting at which the patient fails to distinguish one prong from two prongs.

Check: a random sequence of one or two prongs allows you to assess testing.

- *Normal*: index finger<5 mm; little finger<7 mm; hallux<10 mm.

  N.B. Varies considerably according to skin thickness.
  Compare right with left.

 TIP   It is quite easy to get bogged down testing sensation. Here are some tips for speedy sensory testing:

- Test vibration sense first; then temperature (using the cold of the tuning fork you are holding); then joint position sense; then pinprick. Test light touch last—most time-consuming, least helpful.
- Start distally and work proximally.
- Map any area of sensory loss starting in the area of abnormal sensation then moving towards the normal area.
- Keep a mental drawing of what you have found in mind.

FURTHER TESTS

Sensory inattention
Ask the patient to tell you on which side you touch (either with cotton wool or pinprick). Touch him on the right side and then on the left side. If he is able to recognise each independently, then touch him on both sides at the same time.

What you find
- Recognises right, left and both normally: *normal*.
- Recognises right and left correctly but only one side, usually the right, when both stimulated: *sensory inattention*.

What it means
- Sensory inattention usually indicates a *parietal lobe lesion*, more commonly seen with lesions of the non-dominant hemisphere.

SENSATION: 22

WHAT YOU FIND AND WHAT IT MEANS

WHAT YOU FIND

Patterns of sensory loss

Sensory deficits (Fig. 22.1) can be classified into eight levels of the nervous system:

1. **Single nerve**: sensory loss within the distribution of a single nerve, most commonly median, ulnar, peroneal, lateral cutaneous nerve to the thigh. Distributions are illustrated in Chapter 21.
2. **Root or roots**: sensory deficit confined to a single root or a number of roots in close proximity—common roots in the arm C5, C6 and C7 and in the leg L4, L5 and S1. Distributions are illustrated in Chapter 21. When multiple nerve roots are involved in the lumbosacral spine (usually S1–S5 roots bilaterally), this results in a cauda equina syndrome with sensory loss in the perianal region and buttocks (saddle anaesthesiae) and the back of both thighs.
3. **Peripheral nerve**: distal glove and stocking deficit (Fig. 22.2).
4. **Spinal cord**: five patterns of loss can be recognised (Fig. 22.3):
   - *Complete transverse lesion*: hyperaesthesia (increased appreciation of touch/pinprick) at the upper level, with loss of all modalities a few segments below the lesion (Fig. 22.3A).
   - *Hemisection of the cord* (Brown–Séquard syndrome): loss of joint position sense and vibration sense on the same side as the lesion and pain and temperature on the opposite side a few levels below the lesion (Fig. 22.3B).
   - *Central cord*: loss of pain and temperature sensation at the level of the lesion, where the spinothalamic fibres cross in the cord, with other modalities preserved (dissociated sensory loss)— seen in syringomyelia (Fig. 22.3C).
   - *Posterior column loss*: loss of joint position sense and vibration sense with intact pain and temperature (Fig. 22.3D).
   - *Anterior spinal syndrome*: loss of pain and temperature below the level, with preserved joint position sense and vibration sense (Fig. 22.3E).

Approach to sensory loss

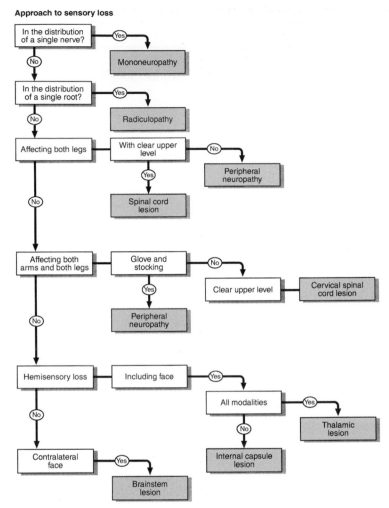

Figure 22.1
Simplified approach to sensory loss

5. **Brainstem**: loss of pain and temperature on the face and on the opposite side of the body. *Common cause*: lateral medullary syndrome (Fig. 22.3F).
6. **Thalamic sensory loss**: hemisensory loss of all modalities (Fig. 22.3G).
7. **Cortical loss**: parietal lobe—the patient is able to recognise all sensations but localises them poorly—loss of two-point discrimination, astereognosis, sensory inattention.
8. **Functional loss**: this diagnosis is suggested by a non-anatomical distribution of sensory deficit frequently with inconstant findings.

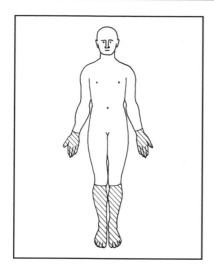

Figure 22.2
Glove and stocking loss

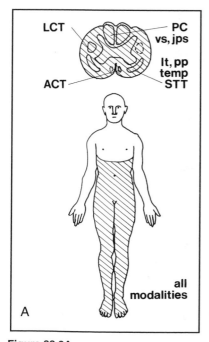

Legend for Figure 22.3 A-G
Cross-section of spinal cord: these are the same as in Figure 21.1, with the lesions shaded in blue. LCT, lateral corticospinal tract; ACT, anterior corticospinal tract; PC, posterior column; STT, spinothalamic tract

Sensory modalities: areas of sensory loss are shaded in blue. Modalities are marked: x, absent; tick, present. pp, pinprick; temp, temperature; vs, vibration sense; jps, joint position sense; lt, light touch

Figure 22.3A
Sensory loss associated with spinal cord lesions: **A.** Complete transverse lesion.

(Continued)

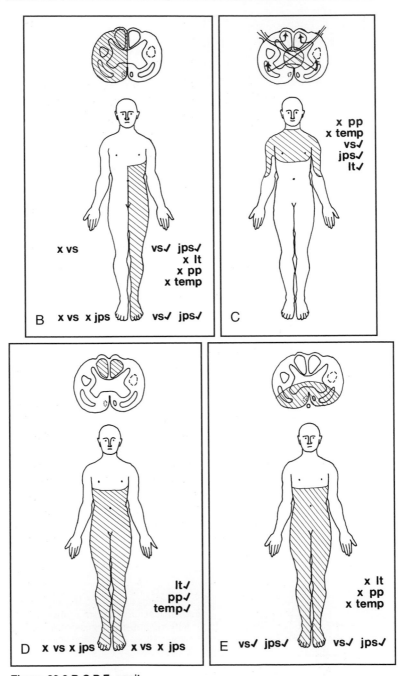

Figure 22.3 B,C,D,E, con't
B. Hemisection of the cord **C.** Central cord lesion. **D.** Posterior column loss.
E. Anterior spinal syndrome

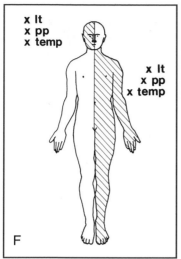
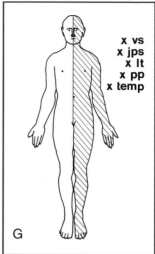

Figure 22.3F,G, con't
F. Brainstem lesion. **G.** Thalamic sensory loss

WHAT IT MEANS

Interpretation of the sensory findings depends on integrating them with the results of other parts of the neurological examination, especially the motor examination.

- **Single nerve lesion.** *Common cause*: entrapment neuropathy. More common in diabetes mellitus, rheumatoid arthritis, hypothyroidism. May be presentation of more diffuse neuropathy (see Chapter 20).
- **Multiple single nerve lesions**: mononeuritis multiplex. *Common causes*: vasculitis, or presentation of more diffuse neuropathy.
- **Single root lesion.** *Common cause*: compression by prolapsed intervertebral discs. *Rare causes*: tumours (e.g. neurofibroma).
- **Cauda equina syndrome** (see also Chapter 26). *Common cause*: compression of cauda equina by prolapsed intervertebral disc. *Rare causes*: tumours or herpes simplex polyradiculitis.
- **Peripheral nerve** (see Chapter 20). *Common causes*: diabetes mellitus, alcohol-related vitamin B_1 deficiency, drugs (e.g. vincristine); frequently no cause is found. *Rarer causes*: Guillain–Barré syndrome, inherited neuropathies (e.g. Charcot–Marie–Tooth disease), vasculitis, other vitamin deficiencies, including vitamin B_{12}.
- **Spinal cord**:
    - **Complete transection.** *Common causes*: trauma, spinal cord compression by tumour (usually bony secondaries in vertebra), cervical spondylitis, transverse myelitis, multiple sclerosis. *Rare*

causes: intraspinal tumours (e.g. meningiomas), spinal abscess, post-infectious (usually viral).
- **Hemisection.** *Common causes*: as for transection.
- **Central cord syndrome** (rare). *Common causes*: syringomyelia, trauma leading to haematomyelia.
- **Posterior column loss**: any cause of complete transection but also the rare subacute combined degeneration of the cord (vitamin B$_{12}$ deficiency) and tabes dorsalis.
- **Anterior spinal syndrome** (rare): anterior spinal artery emboli or thrombosis.
- **Brainstem pattern** (rare). *Common causes*: in young patients—demyelination; in older patients—brainstem stroke. *Rare causes*: brainstem tumours.
- **Thalamic and cortical loss.** *Common causes*: stroke (thrombosis, emboli or haemorrhage), cerebral tumour, multiple sclerosis, trauma.
- **Functional**: may indicate conversion disorder. N.B. This is a difficult diagnosis to make.

 TIP   The diverse range of aetiologies offered for each of the patterns of sensory loss reinforces the importance of the history in making sense of the clinical findings.

23

COORDINATION

BACKGROUND

A coordinated combination of a series of motor actions is needed to produce a smooth and accurate movement. This requires integration of sensory feedback with motor output. This integration occurs mainly in the cerebellum.

In the presence of weakness, tests for coordination must be interpreted with caution and are unlikely to be informative if there is significant weakness.

Loss of joint position sense can produce some incoordination (sensory ataxia). This is made substantially worse when the eyes are closed. Joint position sense should be tested before coordination.

WHAT TO DO

Test the gait (see Chapter 4).

In all tests, compare right with left. Expect the right hand to be slightly better (in a right-handed person).

Arms

Ask the patient to hold his arms outstretched and ask him to close his eyes. Tell the patient to keep his arms in this position. Then push his arm up or down suddenly.

Finger–nose test

Hold your finger out about an arm's length in front of the patient. Ask the patient to touch your finger with his index finger and then touch his nose (Fig. 23.1). When he has done this correctly, ask him to repeat the movement faster. Watch for accuracy and smoothness of movement.

Repeated movements

Ask the patient to pat one hand on the back of the other quickly and regularly (*demonstrate*).

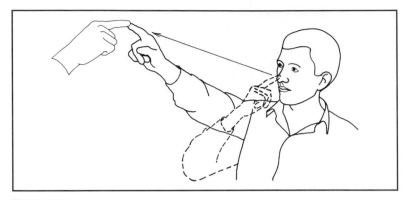

Figure 23.1
The finger–nose test

Ask the patient to twist his hand as if opening a door or unscrewing a light bulb (*demonstrate*).

Ask the patient to tap the back of his right hand alternately with the palm, and then the back of his left hand. Repeat with the right hand (*demonstrate*).

Legs

Heel–shin test

The patient is lying down. Ask him to lift his leg and place the point of his heel on his knee, and then run it down the sharp part of his shin (Fig. 23.2) (*demonstrate*). Watch for accuracy and smoothness of movement.

COMMON MISTAKES

- Do not allow the patient to run his instep along his shin, as this acts as a guide-rail and can mask incoordination.

Ask the patient to tap his feet as if listening to fast music.

Trunk

Ask the patient to sit up from lying without using his hands. Does he fall to one side?

Other tests of cerebellar function

- Speech (Chapter 2).
- Nystagmus (Chapter 10).
- Hypotonia (Chapter 16).
- Pendular reflexes (Chapter 19).
- Tremor (Chapter 24).

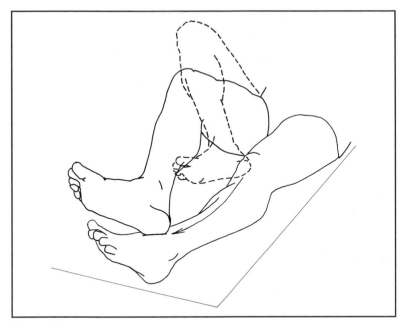

Figure 23.2
The heel–shin test

WHAT YOU FIND

With outstretched arms

- The arms oscillate several times before coming to rest: this indicates *cerebellar disease.*
- The arms return rapidly to position: *normal.*

Finger–nose test

- The patient is able to complete the task quickly and accurately: *normal.*
- The patient develops a tremor as his finger approaches its target: *intention tremor;* finger overshoots its target: *past pointing* or *dysmetria.*

Repeated movements

- Disorganisation of the movement of the hands and the elbows take wider excursions than expected; irregularity of the movements which are performed without rhythm. Compare the two sides; these changes indicate *cerebellar incoordination.* Often the abnormality is heard as a slapping sound rather than the normal tapping noise.

TIP Mild upper motor neurone weakness impairs fluency of fast repeated movements. However, the movements will not have a wider excursion than expected.

When there is disorganisation of tapping the hand and then turning it over, this is referred to as *dysdiadochokinesia*.

Heel–shin test

- Disorganisation of movement with the heel falling off the anterior part of the shin, and the knee falling from side to side.

 TIP The finger–nose and heel–shin tests can be used to test joint position sense. If the movements are accurate with eyes open but are substantially worse when repeated with eyes closed, this indicates impairment of joint position sense.

Trunk

- The patient is unable to sit from lying without falling to one side: *truncal ataxia*. This is associated with gait ataxia (Chapter 4).

WHAT IT MEANS

- **Unilateral incoordination**: ipsilateral cerebellar syndrome.
- **Bilateral incoordination**: bilateral cerebellar syndrome.
- **Truncal ataxia, gait ataxia, without limb incoordination**: midline cerebellar syndrome.
- **Unilateral cerebellar syndrome.** *Common causes*: demyelination, vascular disease. *Rare causes*: trauma, tumour or abscess.
- **Bilateral cerebellar syndrome.** *Common causes*: drugs (anticonvulsants), alcohol, demyelination, vascular disease. *Rare causes*: hereditary cerebellar degenerations, paraneoplastic disorders, hypothyroidism.
- **Midline cerebellar syndrome**: lesion of the cerebellar vermis. *Causes* as for bilateral cerebellar syndrome.

24

ABNORMAL MOVEMENTS

BACKGROUND

Abnormal movements are best appreciated by seeing affected patients. If you are armed with the right vocabulary, most common abnormal movements can be described. However, many experts will describe the same movements in different ways—so journals about movement disorders come with video clips to illustrate the movements!

In most patients with movement disorder, the diagnosis depends on an accurate description of the clinical phenomenon.

There is frequently a considerable overlap between syndromes, and several types of abnormal movement are often seen in the same patient—for example, tremor and dystonia in a parkinsonian patient on treatment.

The anatomy of the basal ganglia is complicated and wiring diagrams illustrating the connections between the various structures become more complicated as more research is done. Neuro-anatomical correlations are of limited clinical value as most movement disorders are classified as syndromes rather than on anatomical grounds. Correlations of significance include unilateral parkinsonism due to lesions of contralateral substantia nigra and unilateral hemiballismus due to lesions of the contralateral subthalamic nucleus or its connections.

In evaluating movement disorders, there are three aspects to the examination:

1. **Positive phenomena**

   – the abnormal positions maintained
   – the additional movements seen.

2. **Latent phenomena**

   – the abnormal phenomena that can be revealed using various manœuvres (e.g. rigidity on testing tone and the abnormal postures brought on by writing in writer's cramp).

3. **Negative phenomena**

   – the inability to do things: for example, a slowness in initiating actions (bradykinesia).

Terms used in movement disorders (Fig. 24.1)

Akathisia: motor restlessness where the patient constantly shifts, crossing and uncrossing his legs and walking on the spot.

Athetosis: slower, writhing, irregular movements predominantly in the hands and wrist (used less frequently now).

Chorea: non-rhythmical movements of a rapid, jerky nature which frequently appear pseudo-purposeful. They may be voluntarily controlled for a short time.

Dyskinesia: a term used to describe movements associated with neuroleptic drugs; particularly used to describe movements of mouth and face (orofacial dyskinesia).

Dystonia: co-contraction of agonist and antagonist which may lead to an intermittent or persistent maintenance of abnormal posture. Position maintained is usually at an extreme of extension or flexion.

Hemiballismus: violent and flinging movements which are irregular, affecting one side. There is no clear distinction from severe chorea.

Myoclonic jerk: an extremely brief contraction of a muscle group leading to involuntary purposeless jerk of the affected limb.

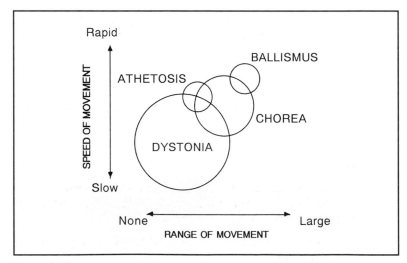

Figure 24.1
There is a considerable overlap between chorea and athetosis; chorea and hemiballismus; and chorea and dystonia

Negative myoclonus: irregular sudden brief loss of muscle tone when a limb is held outstretched. The most common form is asterixis.

Tic: a stereotyped and irresistible repetitive action, normally a repeated purposeful action.

Tremor: rhythmical alternating movement.

WHAT TO DO

Look at the patient's face.

- Are there any additional movements?
- Is the face expressionless?

Look at the patient's head position.
Look at the arms and the legs.

- Note the position.
- Are there any abnormal movements?

Ask the patient to:

- smile
- close his eyes
- hold his hands out in front of him with his wrists cocked back (Fig. 24.2A)
- lift his elbows out sideways and point his index fingers at one another in front of his nose (Fig. 24.2B)
- perform the finger–nose test (as in Chapter 23).

If there is a tremor, note the frequency, the degree of the excursion (fine, moderate, large) and the body parts affected. Look for a tongue tremor (see Chapter 13).

Test eye movements (Chapter 9).
Test tone (Chapter 16).

- When testing tone in one arm, it is sometimes useful to ask the patient to lift the other arm up and down.

Test fast repeating movements.

Ask the patient to:

- bring thumb and index finger rapidly together (*demonstrate*)
- touch the thumb with each finger rapidly in turn (*demonstrate*)
- tap his toe as if listening to fast music.

Observe the speed of the movements and whether they break up; compare right with left.

Test gait (Chapter 4).
Test writing.

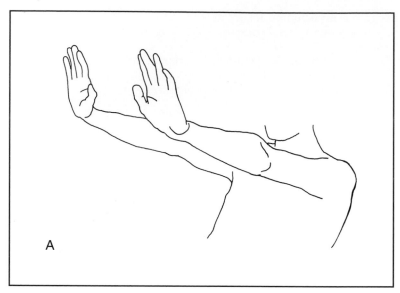

Figure 24.2A
Testing for tremor

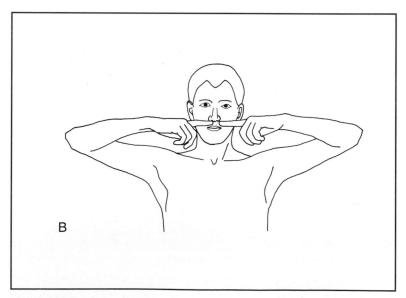

Figure 24.2B
Testing for tremor

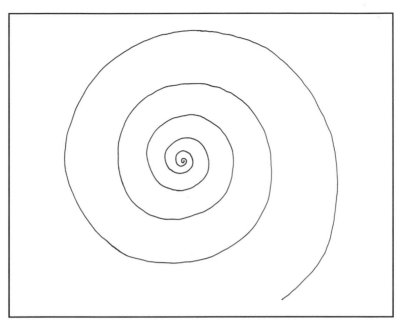

Figure 24.3
Archimedes spiral

Ask the patient to:

- write his name and address
- draw an Archimedes spiral (Fig. 24.3).

Ask the patient to perform any manœuvre that he reports may trigger the abnormal movement.

WHAT YOU FIND

Face

Positive phenomena
Commonly:

- Lip-smacking and twisting of mouth: *orofacial dyskinesia*.
- Flickering of muscles, particularly around eye: *facial myokymia*.

Rarely:

- Intermittent spasm of muscles around the eyes: *blepharospasm*.
- Intermittent spasm of muscles of one side of the face: *hemifacial spasm*.

Negative phenomena
- Facial immobility.

Head

Positive phenomena
Position
- Head twisted to one side: *torticollis*.
- Head leant to one side: *laterocollis*.
- Head bent forward: *anterocollis*.
- Head bent backwards: *retrocollis*.

Movement
- Rhythmical movement of head: *titubation*—described as yes–yes (shaking forward–backwards) or no–no (side to side).

Arms and legs

Positive phenomena
Tremor
- Present when limb (particularly hand) is at rest: *rest tremor*.
- Present when limb is maintained in a position (especially as in Fig. 24.2): *postural tremor*.
- Present during an action (e.g. finger–nose testing): *action tremor*.
- Present and increasing as the finger reaches its target: *intention tremor*.

 TIP Commonly more than one type of tremor coexists.

Asterixis
- Irregular jerky movements of the hands, seen especially in the position illustrated in Figure 24.2. This is actually a sudden loss of tone—*negative myoclonus*.

Position
- Limb maintained, often only transiently, in abnormal position with contraction of both agonists and antagonists: *dystonic posturing*. Commonly the arm is abducted at the shoulder, extended at the elbow, and pronated to an extreme position with the fingers extended. The leg is usually extended at the hip and knee and inverted at the ankle with the toes flexed.

 TIP Try to put yourself into these positions to realise what they look like (and why patients find them uncomfortable).

Additional movements (as described above). Describe which part of the movements are seen to be affected:

- myoclonus
- chorea
- hemiballismus
- tic
- athetosis.

Latent phenomena
On walking, the following may occur or increase:

- rest tremor
- dystonic posturing
- chorea.

Finger–nose testing may reveal:

- action tremor
- intention tremor (see above)
- myoclonus: *action myoclonus*.

and exacerbate:

- choreic movements.

Fast repeating movements
- Slowed or break up easily: *bradykinesia*.

Tone
- Cogwheel rigidity may be found only when the other arm is lifted up and down (activated).

Writing
- Writing becomes progressively slower, the hand may go into spasm, and the patient often holds the pen in an unusual way: writer's cramp.

Archimedes spiral
- Spiral very tight, ending up as a circle: suggests parkinsonism.
- Spiral very large with tremor: suggests cerebellar syndrome essential tremor.

Negative phenomena
- Rigidity: lead pipe or cogwheel.
- Bradykinesia: slowness in initiating movements.
- Reduced arm-swing on walking (see Chapter 4).

WHAT IT MEANS

Akinetic–rigid syndromes (parkinsonism) (common)

- *Key features*: rigidity, bradykinesia and tremor. Features include reduced facial expression (mask-like), rest tremor, stooped posture with reduced arm-swing and increased tremor on walking. Gait may be festinant (see Chapter 4). Bradykinesia on fast repeating movements and walking. Extrapyramidal dysarthria (see Chapter 2). There may be limitation of convergence.
- *Common causes*: Parkinson's disease, antipsychotic drugs, particularly the older agents (e.g. chlorpromazine, haloperidol).
- *Rare causes*: Steele–Richardson syndrome or progressive supranuclear palsy (PSP) (akinetic–rigid syndrome associated with progressive supranuclear palsy), multiple systems atrophy (akinetic–rigid syndrome associated with autonomic failure, pyramidal signs and cerebellar syndrome), Wilson's disease.

Tremors (common)

- **Rest tremor**: feature of akinetic rigid syndrome (see above).
- **Postural and action tremor**: *Common causes*: essential tremor (also called familial tremor if there is a family history), exaggerated physiological tremor (may be caused by hyperthyroidism, beta-agonists). *Rarer causes*: liver failure, renal failure, alcohol withdrawal.
- **Intention tremor**: indicates cerebellar disease (see Chapter 23).

Chorea (uncommon)

Common cause:

- Drug therapy of Parkinson's disease (excess treatment).

Rare causes:

- Wilson's disease (look for associated liver disease and Keyser–Fleischer rings on cornea).
- Huntington's disease (trace family history).
- Post-pill or pregnancy chorea.
- Sydenham's chorea.
- Stroke.

Hemiballismus (rare)

- Lesion of the contralateral subthalamic nucleus or its connections. *Common cause*: stroke.

Dystonia (uncommon)

Affects only one part of the body during a particular action: **task-specific dystonia**

* Isolated writer's cramp.

Affects only one part of the body: **focal dystonia**

* Isolated torticollis.

Affecting two or more adjacent parts of the body: **segmental dystonia.** *For example*:

* Torticollis and dystonic posturing in the same arm.

Affects parts of the body that are not adjacent:

* **Generalised dystonia**: often associated with chorea.

Common causes:

* **Focal and segmental dystonia**: idiopathic, antipsychotic drugs, treated Parkinson's disease on excessive therapy.
* **Generalised dystonia**: as for chorea above.

Rare cause: dystonia musculorum deformans.

Tic (uncommon)

Usually an isolated finding which may be associated with coprolalia (muttering of obscenities); then referred to as Gilles de la Tourette syndrome.

Myoclonic jerk (rare)

May be seen as part of other movement disorders where chorea or dystonia is predominant.

Associated with a number of metabolic encephalopathies, myoclonic epilepsies—seen in rare neurological diseases such as Creutzfeldt–Jakob disease and postanoxic encephalopathy.

Others

* **Orofacial dyskinesia**: usually a late reaction to major tranquilliser. May also occur as part of the syndromes listed under chorea.
* **Akathisia**: late reaction to major tranquilliser.
* **Blepharospasm**: idiopathic.
* **Hemifacial spasm**: compression of facial nerve by ectopic vessels.
* **Facial myokymia**: usually benign, possibly exacerbated by tiredness, caffeine. *Rarely*: indicative of brainstem lesion.
* **Asterixis**: occurs in metabolic encephalopathy, particularly in liver failure.

25

SPECIAL SIGNS AND OTHER TESTS

In this chapter, a number of signs are described which are used on particular occasions:

1. primitive reflexes
2. superficial reflexes
3. tests for meningeal irritation
4. tests of respiratory and trunk muscles
5. miscellaneous tests.

1. PRIMITIVE REFLEXES

Snout reflex

What to do
Ask the patient to close his eyes. Tap his mouth gently with a patella hammer.

What you find
- No reaction: *normal.*
- Puckering of lips: *positive snout reflex.*

Palmo-mental reflex

What to do
Scratch the palm of the patient's hand briskly across the centre of the palm and look at the chin.

What you find
- No reaction: *normal.*
- Contraction of a muscle on the same side of the chin: *positive palmo-mental reflex.*

Grasp reflex

What to do
Place your fingers on the patient's palm and pull your hand away, asking the patient to let go of your hand.

What you find
- The patient is able to let go: *normal*.
- Patient involuntarily grabs your hand: *positive grasp reflex*.

What it means
All these primitive reflexes may be found in normal people. They occur more frequently in patients with frontal pathology and diffuse encephalopathy. If unilateral, they strongly suggest contralateral frontal lobe pathology.

2. SUPERFICIAL REFLEXES

Cremasteric reflex

This reflex can be performed in men. The inner aspect of the upper thigh is stroked downward. The movement of the testicle in the scrotum is watched. Cremasteric contraction elevates the testicle on that side.

- *Afferent*: femoral nerve L1, L2
- *Efferent*: L1, L2.

What you find
- Present: *normal*
- may occur with non-neurological local pathology or previous local surgery
- lesion in reflex arc
- pyramidal lesion above L1.

Anal reflex

What to do
Lie the patient on his side with the knees flexed. Lightly stroke the anal margin with an orange stick.

What you find .
- Visible contraction of the external anal sphincter.

What it means
This tests the integrity of the reflex arc with segmental innervation of S4 and S5 for sensory and motor components. If no contraction seen this indicated a lesion in this reflex arc. Most commonly a cauda equina lesion.

3. TESTS FOR MENINGEAL IRRITATION

Neck stiffness

What to do
N.B. Not to be performed if there could be cervical instability—for example, following trauma or in patients with rheumatoid arthritis.

The patient should be lying flat.

Place your hands behind the patient's head.

- Gently rotate the head, moving the head as if the patient was indicating no. Feel the stiffness.
- Gently lift the head off the bed. Feel the tone in the neck.
- Watch the legs for hip and knee flexion.

What you find and what it means

- Neck moves easily in both planes, with the chin easily reaching the chest on neck flexion: *normal*.
- Neck rigid on movement: *neck stiffness*.
  - Indicates meningeal irritation. *Common causes*: viral and bacterial meningitis, subarachnoid haemorrhage. *Rarer causes*: carcinomatous, granulomatous, fungal meningitis.
  - May also occur in severe cervical spondylosis, parkinsonism, with tonsillar herniation.

  N.B. Proceed to test for Kernig's sign.

- Hip and knee flexion in response to neck flexion: Brudzinski's sign (Fig. 25.1). This indicates meningeal irritation.

> **TIP** Cervical lymphadenopathy and severe pharyngitis may simulate neck stiffness, but stiffness is usually only on flexion and appropriate physical signs of these pathologies are easily found.

Testing for Kernig's sign

What to do

The patient is lying flat on the bed.

- Flex the leg at the hip with the knee flexed.
- Then try to extend the knee.
- Repeat on the other side (Fig. 25.2).

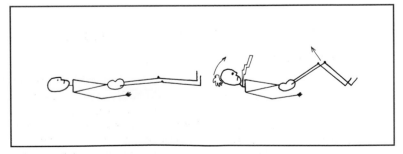

Figure 25.1
Brudzinski's sign

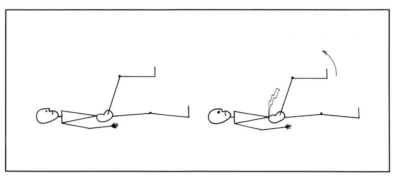

Figure 25.2
Kernig's sign

What you find and what it means
- Knee straightens without difficulty: *normal*.
- Resistance to knee straightening: Kernig's sign—bilateral indicates meningeal irritation; if unilateral, may occur with radiculopathy (cf. straight leg raising).

N.B. Kernig's sign is absent with other causes of neck stiffness.

Head jolt test

A newer sensitive (but not very specific) test for meningeal irritation.

What to do
Ask the patient to turn his head horizontally at a frequency of two or three times a second.

What you find
- No effect: *normal*.
- Worsening of baseline headache: *positive test*.

What it means
- Positive test suggests meningeal irritation is possible.
- Negative test makes meningeal irritation very unlikely.

4. TESTS OF RESPIRATORY AND TRUNK MUSCLES

Respiratory muscles

The intercostal muscles and diaphragm can be involved especially in neuromuscular disorders. Clinical examination can be useful in evaluating respiratory muscle weakness but is of limited value. If respiratory muscle weakness is present, or seriously considered, then physiological measures, particularly vital capacity (which may need to be done lying and standing) and inspiratory mouth pressures, are important and regular monitoring may be needed.

Testing will generally be undertaken if:

- The patient has, or is thought to have, a neuromuscular disorder known to involve respiratory muscles—examples including Guillain–Barré syndrome, myasthenia gravis, motor neurone disease, muscular dystrophy.
- The patient has breathlessness or respiratory failure potentially due to respiratory muscle weakness.

Bedside testing

Is the patient breathless on sitting? Or only on lying flat—when the diaphragm movement is limited by the pressure from the abdominal contents?

Can they talk normally or are they limited to single sentences or only a few words?

Ask them to count—how far can they count on a single breath?

What is the respiratory rate?

Are they using accessory muscles of respiration?

Is the chest expansion normal?

Watch the abdomen—normally the diaphragmatic contraction on inspiration forces the abdomen to go out. If the diaphragm is weak, this is reversed and the abdomen is drawn in on inspiration—paradoxical respiration. This can be unilateral with phrenic nerve palsy.

Axial and trunk muscles

These will be rarely tested formally but are tested indirectly during other elements of the examination—for example when the patient sits up unsupported or walks.

Rarely, patients can present with weakness of axial muscles, for example head drop, when the head hangs forward as a result of weakness of the cervical erector spinae, or camptocormia, when the patient flexes at the waist from weakness of thoracolumbar erector spinae.

Erector spinae can be tested: ask the patient to lie on his front and lift his head up (cervical erector spinae), and then lift his shoulders up (thoracic erector spinae). Then ask him to rest down again and then lift his feet off the couch (lumbar erector spinae).

5. MISCELLANEOUS TESTS AND SIGNS

Tinel's test

Percussion of a nerve at putative site of compression (usually using a tendon hammer). It is positive when paraesthesiae are produced in the distribution of the nerve concerned. Commonly performed to test for median nerve compression at the wrist.

Lhermitte's phenomenon

Forward flexion of the neck produces a feeling of electric shock, usually running down the back. The patient may complain of this spontaneously or you can test for it by flexing the neck. Occasionally, patients have the same feeling on extension (reverse Lhermitte's).

This indicates *cervical pathology*—usually demyelination. It occasionally occurs with cervical spondylitic myelopathy or cervical tumours.

Straight leg raising (Fig. 25.3)

Test for lumbosacral radicular entrapment.

With the patient lying flat on the bed, lift the leg, holding the heel. Note angle attained and any difference between the two sides.

- *Normal* >90 degrees; less in older patients.
- Limitation with pain in back suggests *nerve root entrapment.*

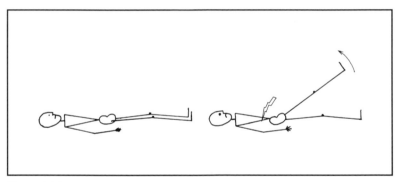

Figure 25.3
Straight leg raising

Head impulse test

The vestibular ocular reflex (VOR) keeps the eyes stable when we move. If it is lacking, our vision jumps up and down like a home-made video (referred to as oscillopsia). The main inputs to this reflex come from the vestibular system in the inner ear and proprioception from the neck muscles. The information is integrated in the brainstem and leads to eye movements to balance the effect of any movement.

The head impulse test is used to examine fast VOR mediated by the lateral semicircular canal and looks at the ability of the eyes to remain stable with rapid movements. It is useful in patients with vertigo.

What to do (Fig. 25.4)

Sit opposite the patient.

Explain that you are going to move his head to look at his balance system and that he will need to relax his neck and let you move his head.

Put your hands on either side of the patient's head.

Ask him to look at a distant object behind your shoulder and to keep looking at that object.

Gently move the head 15 degrees to the right.

(If the patient resists or stiffens the neck, gently move it to the other side, emphasising the need for him to relax, and repeat.)

Then turn the head as rapidly as possible to the left so you end up 15 degrees to the left.

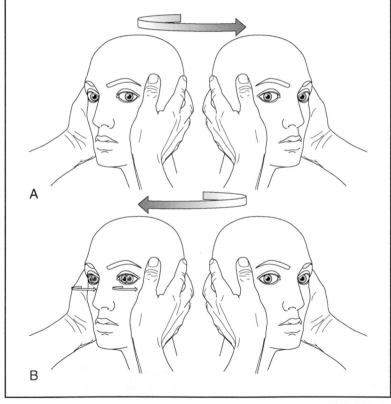

Figure 25.4

Head thrust test. **A.** The patient's head is turned rapidly to his left—note the eyes maintain fixation = normal. **B.** The patient's head is turned rapidly to his right—note the eye has to make a saccade to regain fixation = abnormal right peripheral vestibular system.

Watch the eyes carefully.

Repeat, starting 15 degrees to the left and moving the head to the right.

What you find and what it means

- The eyes remain stable looking at the distant object (Fig. 25.4A): normal VOR.
- The eyes turn with the head and then have to dart back to the correct position to look at the distant vision (a corrective saccade; Fig. 25.4B): indicates a peripheral vestibular lesion on the side the head was moved towards.

The test is highly specific for peripheral vestibular lesions.

Common cause of unilateral peripheral vestibular lesions: vestibular neuritis.

26

THE AUTONOMIC NERVOUS SYSTEM

BACKGROUND

The autonomic nervous system is made up of the sympathetic and parasympathetic nervous systems.

Sympathetic system: ALARM system

Stimulation produces: tachycardia, dilatation of the bronchi, release of adrenaline and noradrenaline (maintains blood pressure), decrease in bowel motility, inhibition of micturition (stimulates internal urethral sphincter, relaxes detrusor muscle), increase in sweating and dilatation of the pupils. (Remember what happens when you go into an exam.)

Parasympathetic system: HOLIDAY system

Stimulation produces: bradycardia, constriction of the bronchi, increase in salivation and lacrimation, increase in bowel motility, erections, initiation of micturition (relaxes the internal urethral sphincter, contraction of detrusor) and constriction of the pupils.

Outflow

- Sympathetic system: T1–L2.
- Parasympathetic system: cranial nerves III, VII, IX and X, and S2–4.

Bedside testing of the autonomic nervous system is limited.
    Patterns of bladder and bowel disturbance are outlined separately (see below).

WHAT TO DO

Examine the pupils (see Chapter 7).
Take the resting pulse.

- Check pulse when asking patients to take 10 breaths per minute.
- Estimate difference between maximum and minimum rate (ideally done using ECG monitoring).

Check pulse response to standing (for 15 beats) (Table 26.1).

Table 26.1
Pulse and BP tests

Test	Normal	Reflex
Resting pulse	60–100	Tachycardia: parasympathetic abnormal
HR response to respiration 10/min	Max–min >15/min	Loss of variation: parasympathetic abnormal
HR response to standing (1st 15 beats)	>11/min increase	Loss of response: parasympathetic abnormal
BP response to standing	Fall <30/15	Increased drop: sympathetic abnormal
HR response to Valsalva	HR up during	HR stable during: sympathetic abnormal
	HR down after	HR stable after: parasympathetic abnormal

HR: heart rate.

Ask the patient to take a deep breath and exhale against a closed glottis: a Valsalva manœuvre (you will probably have to demonstrate this), and then ask him to breathe normally. Note the effect the Valsalva and release have on the pulse.
Take the lying and standing blood pressure (Table 26.1).
Look at the colour of the skin and note any sweating.
Feel the skin temperature.

WHAT YOU FIND

Pupils

- Horner's syndrome (ptosis, miosis, enophthalmos, anhydrosis): *sympathetic defect*.
- Sluggish reactions to light and accommodation: *autonomic neuropathy*.

Skin

- Red and hot with impaired sweating: *sympathetic lesion*.

WHAT IT MEANS

- **Horner's syndrome**: see Chapter 7
- **Autonomic neuropathy**. *Common cause*: diabetes mellitus. *Rare causes*: Guillain–Barré syndrome, amyloidosis, multisystem atrophy

(also called Shy–Drager syndrome: see Chapter 24), orthostatic hypotension, congenital autonomic failure (Riley–Day syndrome).
- **Localised sympathetic lesions**: surgical sympathectomy.

COMMON MISTAKES

- Drugs can interfere with autonomic function tests: e.g. beta-blockers and agents with anticholinergic action block parts of the autonomic nervous system.
- General medical conditions such as pneumonia or anaemia will affect the cardiovascular response and interfere with autonomic testing.

BLADDER AND BOWEL FUNCTION

Patterns of abnormality
Frontal bladder

- Urinary urgency, precipitant and uncontrolled voiding of large volumes without residual urine. Periods of urinary control. Normal anal tone. Frontal release signs (see Chapter 25).
- Occurs in dementia, normal pressure hydrocephalus, frontal tumours.

Spinal bladder

- Initially urinary retention ± overflow incontinence. Later bladder contracts and voids small volumes of urine automatically and precipitantly. Constipation. Normal anal tone. May develop reflex penile erections, called priapism (after the Greek god Priapus).
- Occurs in spinal cord lesions. *Common causes*: trauma, multiple sclerosis. *Rare cause*: spinal tumour.

Peripheral neurogenic bladder

- Painless distension of flaccid bladder with overflow incontinence and large residual volumes. Faecal incontinence. Reduced anal tone. There may be saddle anaesthesia. Impotence.
- Occurs in cauda equina lesions. *Common cause*: central lumbar disc protrusion. *Rarer causes*: spina bifida, ependymomas, cordomas, metastases. Also occurs in peripheral nerve lesions. *Common cause*: diabetes mellitus. *Rarer causes*: pelvic surgery, malignancy.

27

THE UNCONSCIOUS OR CONFUSED PATIENT

BACKGROUND

Level of consciousness: assessment of the unconscious and confused patient

The reticular activating system in the brainstem maintains normal consciousness. Processes that disturb its function will lead to altered consciousness.

This can happen as a result of (Fig. 27.1):

- **diffuse encephalopathy**: generalised disturbance of brain function affecting the whole brain, including the reticular activating system
- **supratentorial lesions**: either massive lesions or those associated with distortion of the brainstem—'coning' (see below)
- **infratentorial lesions**: producing direct damage to the brainstem.

Assessment of patients with altered consciousness will be divided into:

- resuscitation (including some examination to allow you to know how to resuscitate)
- examination.

Examination of unconscious patients must:

- describe in a repeatable way the level of consciousness, so that it can be compared with other observers' results
- distinguish the three syndromes listed above
- attempt to define a cause—frequently requires further investigations.

The terms used to describe levels of unconsciousness—drowsiness, confusion, stuporous, comatose—are part of everyday language and are used in different senses by different observers. It is therefore better to describe the level of consciousness individually in the terms described below. Some issues relating to confusion and delirium are discussed towards the end of the chapter.

Changes in level of consciousness and associated physical signs are very important and need to be monitored. Always record findings.

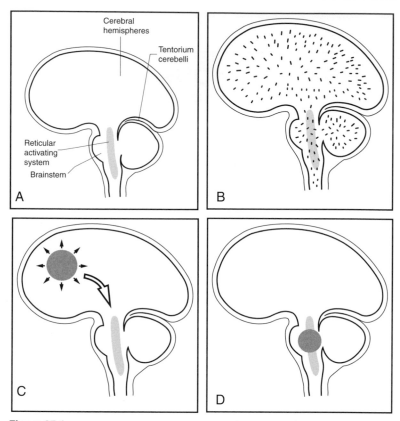

Figure 27.1
Sites of lesions that produce unconsciousness:
A. Key; **B**. Diffuse encephalopathy; **C**. Supratentorial lesions; **D**. Infratentorial lesions

The Glasgow Coma Scale is a quick, simple, reliable method for monitoring level of consciousness. It includes three measures: eye opening, best motor response and best verbal response.

History can be obtained in patients with altered consciousness, from either friends, relatives, bystanders, or nursing or ambulance staff. The clothing (incontinent?), jewellery (alert bracelets/necklaces), wallet and belongings are silent witnesses that may help (Fig. 27.2).

Herniation or coning

Coning is what occurs when part of the brain is forced through a rigid hole, either:

1. the uncus and the temporal lobe through the cerebellar tentorium (which separates the cerebrum from the cerebellum): *uncal herniation;* or

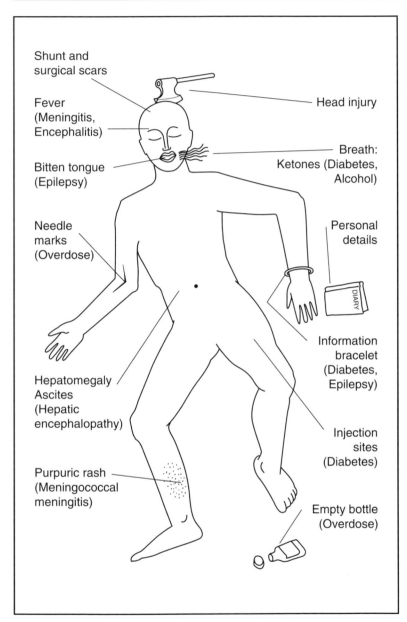

Figure 27.2
Clues to diagnosis in the unconscious patient

2. the cerebrum is pushed centrally through the tentorium: *central herniation*.

There is a characteristic progression of signs in both types of herniation.

> **TIP** The signs of herniation are superimposed on signs due to the supratentorial mass causing the coning, and are progressive.

1. Uncal herniation
What happens
A unilateral mass forces the ipsilateral temporal lobe through the tentorium, compressing the ipsilateral third nerve and later the contralateral upper brainstem, and eventually the whole brainstem. Once cerebrospinal fluid (CSF) flow is interrupted, the process is accelerated by an increase in intracranial pressure.

Physical signs
Early:

- ipsilateral dilated pupil and signs of supratentorial mass lesion.

Later:

- ipsilateral hemiplegia
- progressive ptosis and third nerve palsy
- Cheyne–Stokes respiration.

Later still:

- tetraparesis
- bilateral fixed dilated pupils
- erratic respiration
- death.

Progression is usually rapid.

2. Central herniation
What happens
A supratentorial lesion forces the diencephalon (the thalamus and related structures that lie between the upper brainstem and cerebral hemispheres) centrally through the tentorium. This compresses first the upper midbrain, and later the pons and medulla.

Physical signs
Early:

- erratic respirations
- small reactive pupils

- increased limb tone
- bilateral extensor plantars.

Later:

- Cheyne–Stokes respiration
- decorticate rigidity.

Later still:

- fixed dilated pupils
- decerebrate posturing.

Progression is usually slower.

WHAT TO DO
Resuscitation

Use the Neurological ABC:

N: *Neck*	Always remember there may be a neck injury. If this is possible, do not manipulate the neck.
A: *Airway*	Ensure there is an adequate airway, best protected by putting the patient in the recovery position.
B: *Breathing*	Ensure the patient is breathing sufficiently to provide adequate oxygenation (including blood gases if necessary). Give oxygen and artificial respiration if needed.
C: *Circulation*	Check there is adequate circulation; check pulse and blood pressure.
D: *Diabetes*	Check the blood sugar—Destrostix, BM sticks; if not available, give 50ml 50% dextrose if the altered consciousness could be due to hypoglycaemia.
D: *Drugs*	Consider opiate overdose; give naloxone if indicated.
E: *Epilepsy*	Observe for seizures or stigmata, bitten tongue; control seizures.
F: *Fever*	Check for fever, stiff neck, purpuric rash of meningococcal meningitis.
G: *Glasgow Coma Scale*	Assess score out of 15 (Table 27.1). Record subscores (eyes/verbal/motor) as well as total.
H: *Herniation*	Is there evidence of coning? See above, rapid neurosurgical assessment.
I: *Investigate*	

N.B. Pulse, BP, respiration rate and pattern, temperature. Monitor Glasgow Coma Scale.

Table 27.1
Glasgow Coma Scale

	Score
Eyes open	
Spontaneously	4
To verbal stimuli	3
To pain	2
Never	1
Best verbal response	
Orientated and converses	5
Disorientated and converses	4
Inappropriate words	3
Incomprehensible words	2
No response	1
Best motor response	
Obeys commands	6
Localises pain	5
Flexion—withdrawal to pain	4
Abnormal flexion (decorticate rigidity) (Fig. 27.3A)	3
Abnormal extension (decerebrate rigidity) (Fig. 27.3B)	2
No response	1
Total	**15**

EXAMINATION

This is aimed at:

- finding or excluding focal neurological abnormalities
- looking for evidence of meningism
- determining the level of consciousness and neurological function.

Position and movement

What to do
Look at the patient: often best done from the end of the bed.

- Is the patient lying still or moving?

If there is movement:

- Are all four limbs moved equally?
- Is the patient lying symmetrically?
- Are there any abnormal movements?

What you find
- Arms flexed at elbow and wrist, and legs extended at knee and ankle: *decorticate posturing* (Fig. 27.3A).
- Arms extended at elbow, pronated and flexed at wrist, and legs extended at knee and ankle: *decerebrate posturing* (Fig. 27.3B).
- Head falls to one side, with flexion of the arm: indicates *hemiparesis.*
- There are brief spasms, lasting less than a second, of arms or legs: *myoclonus.*

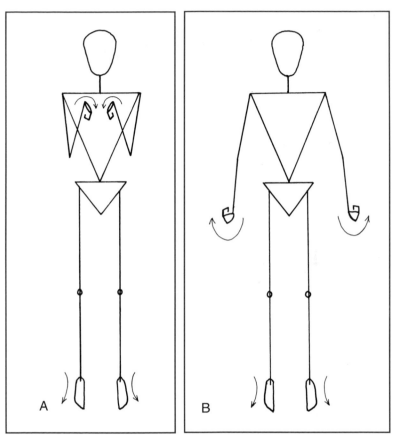

Figure 27.3
Abnormal posturing: **A.** Decorticate; **B.** Decerebrate

Best verbal responses

What to do
Try to rouse the patient.

- Is the patient rousable?

Ask a simple question: 'What is your name?'

If you get a reply:

See if he is oriented:

- In **time**: What day is it? What is the date? What is the month, year? What is the season? What is the time of day?
- In **place**: What is the name of the place we are in? What is the name of the ward/hospital? What is the name of the town/city?
- In **person**: What is your name? What job does that person do (pointing to a nurse)? What job do I do?

Make a note of the errors made.

If you get no reply:

- Try other questions: 'What happened to you?', 'Where do you live?' Note responses.

What you find
Note best level of response:

- oriented
- confused conversation: using long or short sentences
- inappropriate words
- incomprehensible sounds
- none.

COMMON MISTAKES

Aphasia, either receptive or expressive, may be missed—giving a false level of consciousness and missing a focal dominant hemisphere sign (see Chapter 2).

Head and neck

What to do and what you find
- Inspect the head for evidence of trauma.
- Percuss the skull (as for chest percussion): a fracture may be associated with a 'cracked pot sound'.
- Look at the ears and nose for evidence of CSF or bleeding. Examine the eardrums for evidence of otitis media.
- Test the neck for stiffness (see Chapter 25).

If there is evidence of trauma, do not test until cervical injury is excluded.

Eyelids

What to do and what you find
Look at the eyelids.

- Do they open and close spontaneously?
- Tell the patient to open/close his eyes.
- Assess response to pain—do the eyes close?
- Is there any eyelid movement?

Is the eyelid movement symmetrical?

- Is there a ptosis?
- Is there a facial weakness?

Pupils

What to do
Look at the pupils.

- Note size in millimetres.
- Test direct and consensual light reflexes (see Chapter 7).

What you find
See Table 27.2.

Table 27.2
Examining the pupils

Equal?	Size?	Reactive?	Disorder
Pupils equal	Pinpoint		*Opiates or pontine lesion*
	Small	Reactive	*Metabolic encephalopathy*
	Mid-sized	Fixed	*Midbrain lesion*
		Reactive	*Metabolic lesion*
Pupils unequal	Dilated	Unreactive	*Third nerve palsy; N.B. herniation*
	Small	Reactive	*Horner's syndrome*

Fundi

Examine the fundi (Chapter 8).
Look especially for optic nerve head swelling (rare) or subhyaloid haemorrhages.

COMMON MISTAKES

- Absence of papilloedema does not exclude raised intracranial pressure.

Eye movements

What to do
Watch the eye movements.

- Do they look at you?
- Do they follow a moving object, such as a torch?
- Do they move together (conjugately) or independently (disconjugately)?
- Do they move at all?
- What is their position?

Test doll's eye manœuvre (see below).

What you find

- Skew deviation: brainstem lesion.

If the patient can follow objects:

- Test eye movements as in Chapter 9.
- Evidence of III, IV or VI nerve palsies, lateral gaze palsy (see Chapter 9 and consider uncal herniation).

Caloric test: see Chapter 12.
Corneal reflex: see Chapter 11.
Gag reflex: see Chapter 13.

OCULOCEPHALIC TESTING OF EYE MOVEMENTS (DOLL'S EYE MANŒUVRE)

What to do
(N.B. Not to be done unless cervical injury is excluded.)

Turn the head to the right.
Watch the eyes.

- Do they both turn to the left?
- Do they keep looking ahead?
- Does one move and not the other?

Test the other side; text neck extension and flexion.

What you find
- Eyes move in the opposite direction to head movement— as if trying to look straight: *normal*.
- Eyes move to one side but not the other: *lateral gaze palsy*—brainstem lesion.
- Limitation of abduction of one eye: *VI nerve palsy*.
- Limitation of movements other than abduction in one eye with dilated pupil: *III nerve palsy*.
- Eyes fail to move in any direction: *bilateral brainstem lesions*.

Motor system

What to do
Assess the tone in all four limbs (see Chapter 16).

- Is it symmetrical?

Assess the movement in each limb.
Look at the spontaneous movements of the limbs.

- Are they symmetrical?

Ask the patient to move the limb.

If he cooperates: test power more formally.
If no response:

> **Press the knuckle of your thumb into the sternum**.
>
> – Is there a purposeful movement to the site of pain?
> – Do arms flex with this pain?
> – Do arms and legs extend with pain?
> – Is there asymmetry in these responses?

If no response to this stimulus:

> **Apply pressure to inner end of eyebrow**. Note response.
> **Squeeze the nail bed of a digit in each limb**: does limb withdraw?

Tendon reflexes
See Chapter 19.
Are they symmetrical?

Plantar response: extensor or flexor.

What you find
- Best motor response is found:
  - obeys commands
  - localises
  - withdraws
  - abnormal flexion
  - extension response
  - none.
- Record abnormal responses for each limb.
- Asymmetry in tone, reflexes or response to pain: indicates *hemiparesis*.

WHAT YOU FIND AND WHAT IT MEANS

Patients with coma can be classified into one of the following groups:

1. Patients without focal signs
   a. without signs of meningism
   b. with meningism.
2. Patients with focal signs indicative of either central herniation or uncal herniation (supratentorial lesions).
3. Patients with brainstem signs not indicative of coning (infratentorial lesions).

In most patients, accurate diagnosis depends on appropriate further investigations. These investigations are given in parentheses for the Common Causes of Coma.

> ✔ **TIP** Locked-in syndrome: very rarely, patients with a
> midbrain lesion (usually a stroke) can become 'locked in'.
> They are awake and aware but the only movement under
> voluntary control is moving their eyes upwards—limiting
> communication. However, they will look up if you ask
> them to (but only if you do—so think about the diagnosis).

COMMON CAUSES OF COMA

The most common are marked with an asterisk.

1. Diffuse and multifocal processes

a. Without meningism
Metabolic
- *Hypoglycaemia (blood glucose).
- *Hyperglycaemia (blood glucose).
- *Hypoxia (blood gases).
- *Acidosis (blood gases).
- Thiamine deficiency, 'Wernicke's encephalopathy'.
- Hepatic failure.
- Renal failure.
- Hypercapnia (excess CO_2).
- Hypoadrenalism.

Toxin-induced
- **Drugs: benzodiazepines, barbiturates, opiates, tricyclics (toxicology screen).
- *Alcohol (toxicology).

Infectious
- *Encephalitis: herpes simplex and other viruses (CSF examination, EEG).

Vascular
- Hypertensive encephalopathy.

Trauma
- *Concussion (CT or MRI brain scan).
- Fat emboli.

Epilepsy
- *Post-ictal.

Temperature regulation
- Hypothermia (rectal temperature).

b. With meningism
Vascular
- *Subarachnoid haemorrhage (CT brain, CSF examination). N.B. May have focal signs: brainstem or hemisphere.

Infectious
- Meningitis: bacterial and viral (blood cultures, CT or MRI brain scan, CSF examination and culture).

2. Supratentorial lesions (CT or MRI brain scan)

- Haemorrhage
  - Extradural
  - *Subdural
  - *Intracerebral.
- Infarction
  - Embolic
  - Thrombotic.
- Tumours
  - Primary
  - Secondary.
- Abscess.
- Hydrocephalus
  - Including blocked shunt.

3. Infratentorial lesions (CT or MRI brain scan)

- Haemorrhage
  - Cerebellar
  - Pontine.
- Infarction
  - Brainstem.
- Tumours
  - Cerebellum.
- Abscess
  - Cerebellum.

THE CONFUSED PATIENT—DELIRIUM

Some additional comments on patients with confusion or delirium.

Background

The cardinal features of delirium (or acute confusional state) are:

- recent onset
- impaired attention
- disordered thinking.

Patients may be apathetic or agitated and have delusions or hallucinations (often visual).

Delirium occurs with a diffuse encephalopathy (see Fig. 27.1B)—a process that leads to unconsciousness—coma—if more severe. This can arise from a wide range of causes (see later).

Delirium occurs more often in patients with a pre-existing cognitive deficit—and in those patients can arise with less severe provocation.

Patients with confusion are often difficult to assess; an approach is outlined here.

History will be limited. Obtain what information you can from witnesses, family members or members of staff—particularly about usual level of function and of anything to suggest a pre-existing cognitive deficit.

 TIP   Think 'one hit or two?'

A patient with prior brain disorder (hit 1) requires a less significant insult (hit 2) to become confused. Indeed, patients with significant pre-existing brain disorders (such as mild dementia) can become very confused with a systemic upset that does not primarily involve the brain— such as a chest or urinary infection.

Someone with a previously healthy brain requires a more significant insult to the brain (hit 1) to cause confusion.

What to do

A complete general and neurological examination may be impossible if the patient will not co-operate—in which case, it is worth focusing on the most important elements.

Check pulse, blood pressure, respiratory rate and glucose.
Look for signs of infection on general examination.
Check for neck stiffness.

Observe behaviour (see Chapter 3).
Assess orientation in time, place and person (see Chapter 3).
Check attention and concentration—using digit span and serial sevens.
Use simple tests for memory.
If possible, check visual fields, eye movement, fundoscopy, facial symmetry, power in all four limbs, reflexes and plantar response. Sensory testing is likely to be limited.

What you find

- Patients may be agitated or apathetic with impaired attention and short-term memory.
- They may have signs of infection (especially important if prior neurological disorder):
  - Non-specific—fever, tachycardia
  - Non-neurological infection—for example, signs of chest infection or
  - Neurological infection—purpuric rash, neck stiffness.
- They may have stigmata of other general medical disorder (see Fig 27.2).
- They may have neck stiffness—meningism.

What it means

All the diffuse and metabolic processes and supratentorial causes of coma (pages 204–5) can cause delirium. Some conditions such as alcohol withdrawal will cause confusion but not coma.

In addition, in patients with pre-existing cognitive deficits, a modest second pathology, particularly systemic infection—urinary tract infections or pneumonia—can present with delirium. Conversely, a systemic infection is much less likely to explain confusion in a patient who was previously normal.

The diagnosis of the cause of delirium depends on prompt further investigation.

A useful mnemonic to remind you of common reversible causes of delirium is WHIP TIME:

W—Wernicke's encephalopathy and withdrawal from alcohol
H—hypoglycaemia, hypoxia, hypertension
I—ictal (epilepsy)
P—poisoning
T—trauma
I—intracranial haemorrhage
M—meningitis
E—encephalitis.

28

SUMMARY OF STANDARD NEUROLOGICAL EXAMINATION

If the history provides no suggestion of focal neurological deficit, no speech disturbance and no disturbance of higher function, then you can use a standard neurological examination. If you find any abnormality or if the history points to a likely deficit, then that must be explored further.

Standard neurological examination

- **Gait**.
- **Pupils**: direct and consensual reactions.
- **Test fields** to hand movements.
- **Fundoscopy**.
- **Eye movements** to pursuit on upgaze and lateral gaze.
- **Facial sensation** to light touch with fingertip in all three divisions of trigeminal.
- **Facial movement**: 'Screw up your eyes—show me your teeth.'
- **Mouth**: 'Open your mouth' (look at tongue) 'and say "ahh"' (observe palate). 'Please put out your tongue.'
- Test neck flexion.
- **Arms**:
  - Look for wasting.
  - Test tone at wrist and elbow.
  - Observe outstretched arms with eyes closed (pronator test).
  - Test power (shoulder abduction, elbow flexion and extension, finger extension and abduction and abductor pollicis brevis).
- **Legs**:
  - Look for wasting.
  - Test tone at hip.
  - Test power (hip flexion and extension, knee flexion and extension, foot dorsiflexion and plantarflexion).
- **Reflexes**:
  - Test reflexes in arms and legs (biceps, triceps, supinator knee, ankle and plantar response).

- **Sensation**:
    - Test joint position sense in toes and fingers.
    - Test vibration sense on toes and fingers.
    - Test light touch and pinprick distally in hands and feet.
- **Coordination**: test finger–nose and heel–shin.

29

PASSING CLINICAL EXAMINATIONS

BACKGROUND

Clinical examinations come in all shapes and sizes. Most medical students focus on their licensing or 'final' exams, doctors in training on exams testing further skills, such as the MRCP, or those that provide specialist status, such as the Boards in the United States.

The examiners in all these examinations have the same objective: to test the candidates' competence in areas that are important in clinical practice. In devising the examination format, the examiners are aware that:

- the situation is artificial
- the test should be consistent and fair
- many candidates will 'learn for the exam'.

Thus, examiners continually amend the format of the examination so that it is more valid, more reliable and more closely aligned to clinical practice. Currently the trend is away from 'spot diagnosis' to an observation of limited focused clinical examination. This aims to replicate what happens clinically, and to encourage candidates to learn the skills they will need in practice.

These examinations have differing formats but almost all include a requirement for the candidate to perform the following stages:

- **Stage 1**: Examine a patient neurologically, observed by an examiner.[1] The examiner will be looking for a *systematic, appropriate* and *thorough* neurological examination, using *reliable* examination technique. They will also observe for *communication skills,* including rapport with the patient, *professional manner* and treating the patient with appropriate consideration and empathy. In other words, 'what you do'.
- **Stage 2**: Describe the findings, coming to some sort of conclusion.[1] The examiner will be looking for a *correct identification of abnormal physical signs,* an *appropriate interpretation* of these abnormalities,

---

[1] These are the three elements on the examiner's mark sheet for the neurological part of PACES in MRCP.

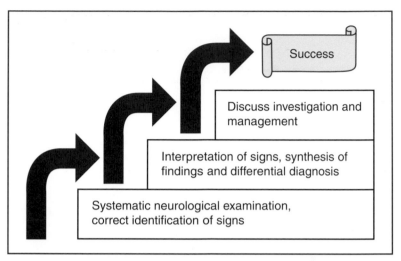

Figure 29.1
Three steps to success

and a *reasonable synthesis* of the findings and suggested diagnoses and differential diagnosis. In other words, 'what you find' and 'what it means'. Interpreting the signs depends on getting the signs right and this will depend on having done the examination properly—so stage 2 depends on stage 1.

- **Stage 3**: Discuss the further investigation or management of the patient's problem.[1] The examiner will discuss aspects of further investigation and management. This tests the candidate's knowledge relating to this particular clinical problem. This is not the focus of the clinical part of the examination, as this knowledge is often tested using other examination formats. Discussing these elements further depends on having an appropriate diagnosis or differential diagnosis—so stage 3 depends on stage 2, which depends on stage 1 (Fig. 29.1).

Most candidates run into problems with stages 1 and 2, and may not get to stage 3. The examiners may try to help, with prompting or leading questions (let them).

The best way to pass the exam is to be competent. This is why this chapter is at the end of the book. So, if you turned straight to this section, go right back to the beginning of the book (unless it's an emergency[2]).

WHAT TO DO

Consider each stage of the examination in turn.

---

[2] See last part of this section: Learning neurological examination in a crisis.

Stage 1: Examine a patient neurologically, observed by an examiner

You are not meant to reach a stunning diagnosis but to demonstrate that your examination is:

- systematic
- practised
- reliable
- appropriate
- thorough
- professional.

The difficulties arise because:

- you are unable to undertake a systematic, practised, reliable, appropriate and thorough examination
- time is limited
- you are anxious (especially if the first point is true).

The solution is to sort out the first point; when competent at examination, you will use time more efficiently and become confident.

Systematic, practised and reliable

This book is set out to allow you to develop a systematic approach to clinical examination using reliable methods.

To develop a system you can rely on, you need to practise. Professional golfers practise hitting the ball thousands of times on the driving range so when under pressure in competition they know just what to do. Neurological examination is just the same. What you need to do has been described throughout the book; the more you do it and the quicker you become, the less you are concerned about what you should do next and the more confident you are in your findings being normal or abnormal. Generally speaking, you will also look slicker.

Practising with someone watching you can help this further—preferably someone more experienced, but colleagues can also help. Think about 'demonstrating' physical signs so that your spectator will also see any abnormalities you find. You can learn by watching—anyone; you often learn as much watching someone having difficulties doing something as watching an expert. You will also be less anxious in the exam if you are used to being watched.

Appropriate and thorough

In some clinical examinations you are asked to do only a partial examination and are usually provided with only a limited history: for example, 'Please examine this man, who has had progressive difficulty walking over the last year.' This is not as artificial as it seems. In clinical practice most patients will have one problem that will be the focus of the neurological examination and the rest of the neurological examination is effectively a screening examination. You should therefore be able to work out what is 'appropriate' in the context of the exam (Table 29.1). It is useful to think of 'appropriate' in this context as 'what is needed to solve the clinical problem'.

A systematic examination that is appropriate will inevitably be thorough; that is, it will cover all the necessary parts of the examination. It does not have to be obsessional or fussy to be thorough; indeed, this would waste valuable time.

Professional

Be polite, courteous and considerate—as you should be with all patients (and colleagues!).

Table 29.1
Some common clinical problems seen in examinations

Clinical problem	Focused examination	Common syndromes
Walking difficulties	Gait Motor system; tone, power; reflexes Sensation Coordination Consider: fast repeating movements; eye movements; speech	Cerebellar syndrome Akinetic rigid syndrome Spastic paraparesis (with or without sensory signs) Peripheral neuropathy
Numb hands and feet and loss of dexterity	Gait Motor system; tone, power; reflexes Sensation Coordination	Spastic tetraparesis with sensory signs Peripheral neuropathy
Weakness in arms and legs	Gait Motor system; tone, power; reflexes Sensation Coordination	Spastic tetraparesis with or without sensory signs Mixed upper and lower motor neurone syndrome Peripheral neuropathy
Speech difficulties	Speech Face Mouth	Dysarthria Dysphonia Aphasia (less likely)
Double vision	Eye movements	Cranial nerve lesion VI, III or IV Myasthenia gravis Thyroid eye disease
Visual problems	Acuity Fields Fundi Possibly eye movements	Optic atrophy Homonymous hemianopia Bitemporal hemianopia

COMMON MISTAKES

- Not thinking. Remember you are trying to solve a clinical problem.
- Rushing into the examination and not looking at the whole patient. You may fail to observe simple things like pes cavus or scars. If you are examining the eyes of a patient in a wheelchair, it is likely the eye problem has something to do with the mobility problem—a helpful clue.
- Worrying about the ritual of the examination. Remember, neurological examination is a tool to help you test how the nervous system is functioning and in what way it is not functioning. It is not a dance.
- Forgetting what you have found. It is useful to summarise your findings in your head as you go along; this helps ensure you are thorough, as you should recognise any gaps that need filling.
- Getting bogged down with sensory testing. This commonly happens if you start by testing light touch, and test proximally to distally. To avoid this, test vibration sense, then proprioception, then pinprick and temperature. Start testing distally and work proximally (see Chapters 21 and 22).
- Finding signs that are not there. If there is something you are not sure about, examine it again. Generally it is worse to find something that is not there than to miss something that is. Remember, it is perfectly reasonable to be asked to examine a patient with no neurological abnormalities. (There may be clues in the history: 'Please examine this man, who has *intermittent* walking problems' (my italics).)
- Forgetting what you would do in the real world. If, for example, you found that sensory testing was not adequate because of time, say so. 'Sensory testing was limited by time and I would be keen to repeat it.' However, generally, patients will have been selected so that an adequate assessment can be undertaken in the time available.
- Examining the left eye with the ophthalmoscope and eliciting the left ankle reflex are particularly difficult and need practice to perfect—so examiners watch you do these with great interest!

Stage 2: Describe your findings, coming to some sort of conclusion

The examiners will have watched you examine the patient and will have a reasonable idea of what you have found (demonstrated). They will ask you to describe your findings or conclusions—remember to answer the question they ask. How you answer will also depend on the level of the exam you are taking. There are three approaches:

1. To describe the physical signs systematically (A), using the conventional order, summarising them (B), then coming to a synthesis of the signs (C) and suggested differential diagnoses (D)—as in Boxes 29.1 and 29.2. This is long-winded, but allows you to describe the physical signs and your reasoning. This approach is generally restricted to final medical student examinations.

BOX 29.1   SYNTHESISING YOUR FINDINGS AND ANSWERING QUESTIONS ON DIAGNOSIS

Example 1 (a relatively complicated case)
Different approaches (see text) describing a patient after a limited examination of the legs of a 'patient with leg weakness'. He looks as if he is aged between 40 and 50.

(A) (*Signs*) The patient was unable to walk. The tone in the right leg was increased, with spasticity at the knee and clonus at the right ankle. The tone in the left leg was normal. There was pyramidal weakness in the right leg, hip flexion grade 2, hip extension grade 2, knee extension grade 3, flexion grade 2, foot dorsiflexion grade 1 and plantar flexion grade 3. The power in the left leg was normal. The tendon reflexes in the right leg were pathologically brisk with an extensor right plantar; the left-sided reflexes were normal with a flexor plantar. There was loss of vibration sense in the right leg to the anterior superior iliac spine, loss of joint position sense in the toes, and reduced proprioception at the knee. The left-sided vibration sense and joint position sense were normal. Pinprick and temperature were lost in the left leg to a sensory level at the costal margin. These modalities were normal in the right leg. Coordination was not tested on the right because of weakness; on the left it appeared normal.

(B) (*Summary of signs*) The combination of a right-sided upper motor neurone lesion at or above L1, and a right-sided posterior column sensory loss with a left-sided spinothalamic sensory loss and a sensory level at T8 indicate.

(C) (*Synthesis*) A partial hemicord syndrome (a Brown–Séquard syndrome) at or above T8.

(D) The *differential diagnosis* is of a spinal lesion at or above T8 (*anatomical diagnosis*). This could result from external

BOX 29.1 SYNTHESISING YOUR FINDINGS AND ANSWERING QUESTIONS ON DIAGNOSIS—cont'd

compression or trauma to the spinal cord or an intrinsic lesion within the cord (*pathological diagnosis*). External compression most commonly occurs from disc disease, spondylosis or tumours,* most commonly bony secondaries, though also meningiomas or neurofibromas. Intrinsic lesions are most commonly due to demyelination, either myelitis or related to multiple sclerosis;* more rarely, vascular lesions such as cord infarcts can produce this problem (though typically they produce anterior cord syndromes) or very rarely intrinsic spinal cord tumours.

*See 'N.B. Euphemisms' in text.

BOX 29.2 SYNTHESISING YOUR FINDINGS AND ANSWERING QUESTIONS ON DIAGNOSIS

Example 2 (a relatively straightforward case)
Different approaches (see text) describing a patient after a limited examination of a 'patient with walking difficulties'.

(A) (*Signs*) His gait is abnormal. He is slightly stooped; his gait is narrow-based with small steps. His right arm is slightly flexed and does not swing. His facial expression is reduced. He has a rest tremor in his right hand. He has cogwheel rigidity in the right arm and leg. Power is full. The reflexes are slightly increased on the right. The plantars are flexor. Sensation is normal. There is moderate right-sided bradykinesia, evident on fast repeating movements of hand and foot. Coordination is accurate, though slow on the right.

(B) (*Summary of signs*) This man has a parkinsonian gait and a right-sided rest tremor, with cogwheel rigidity and bradykinesia.

(C) (*Synthesis*) This man has an asymmetrical akinetic rigid syndrome.

(D) (*Differential diagnosis*) The most common cause of an asymmetrical akinetic rigid syndrome is idiopathic Parkinson's disease. Other differential diagnoses to consider are drug-induced parkinsonism (which is usually symmetrical), or rare extrapyramidal diseases such as multisystem atrophy, diffuse Lewy body disease, progressive supranuclear palsy (or, in a young patient, Wilson's disease).

2. To summarise the relevant abnormal signs (B), a synthesis of the signs (C) and suggested differential diagnosis (D)—as in Boxes 29.1 and 29.2. This is more succinct and gives the opportunity to discuss and clarify signs before coming to a synthesis. If these are not quite right, the examiner may wish to prompt you towards the correct interpretation.
3. To propose a synthesis of the signs (C), with or without reference to abnormal signs (± B), and discuss a differential diagnosis (D)—as in Boxes 29.1 and 29.2. However, if signs or synthesis are incorrect, it is more difficult for the examiner to prompt with questions.

Approach 2 is probably the correct strategy in postgraduate examinations if no specific question is asked.

It is worthwhile practising each of these approaches when you see patients and actually to say them out loud—preferably to a more senior colleague; a contemporary will also be able to offer advice. If no one else is there, do it anyway, to practise putting your thoughts into words.

When coming to a synthesis, describe the anatomical or syndromic diagnosis first. Then offer a differential diagnosis of potential causes. You can classify potential causes according to their pathological process rather than specific diseases. Start with common causes; if you suggest a rare cause you might want to tell the examiners you appreciate that it is rare. The examiners are interested in your clinical reasoning, so part of the test is to see how you approach the differential diagnosis.

N.B. Euphemisms: If the discussion occurs while the patient is there, you will be expected to use euphemisms for diagnoses you discuss that are potentially alarming for the patient (especially if they have something else). Examples include: *demyelination* for multiple sclerosis; *anterior horn cell disease* for amyotrophic lateral sclerosis (motor neurone disease); *neoplasia* for cancer.

COMMON MISTAKES

- You fail to answer the question asked. This often involves answering a similar but different question. This is popular with politicians in interviews, but unpopular with examiners.
- When asked about causes of problems, you jump to rare and unlikely pathological diagnoses. Avoid this by starting with an anatomical or syndromic diagnosis and then suggest pathologies, starting with common diseases and then moving on to rarer problems.
- You panic. Sometimes (well, quite often) people get so flustered in exams that they do not do as well as they should. You can avoid this by practising both neurological examination and being in a stressful situation. Presenting cases at clinical meetings or simply asking questions in meetings or lectures provides useful practice in articulating your thoughts under stress.

> **TIP** Here is a helpful way to learn neurology. If you have not seen a patient with a particular disease, then turn the textbook descriptions into descriptions of imaginary patients with appropriate physical signs. This not only helps you remember and recognise the conditions but also helps you practise putting it into words. You can do this anywhere, in the bath or on the bus (though best not say it out loud then!).

Some common or important conditions you might want to practise on are:

- multiple sclerosis
- amyotrophic lateral sclerosis (motor neurone disease)
- cervical radiculomyelopathy
- hereditary motor and sensory neuropathy
- dominant hemisphere middle cerebral artery stroke
- lateral medullary syndrome
- Brown–Séquard syndrome (Box 29.1)
- myotonic dystrophy
- Parkinson's disease (Box 29.2).

Stage 3: Discuss the further investigation or management of the patient's problem

This part of the clinical exam primarily aims to test whether you are sensible and have good 'clinical sense', and does not depend on a wealth of knowledge (though this will help). Knowledge is tested more extensively in other parts of your exams.

Remember that this examination is trying to replicate real clinical practice—so do what you would do in real life. If you have only had a limited history and been able to do a partial neurological examination, you would normally take a full history and complete examination. Suggest this, but indicate what particular aspects you would focus on; for example, in a patient with a neuropathy you might suggest that you would be interested in general medical history, drug or toxin exposure, alcohol intake and detailed family history.

If you are asked about other investigations, indicate how you would use the investigations to solve the clinical problem—why would you do each test? Remember the tests are there to help you—how would they help you?

When suggesting investigations, generally start with the simple ones. However, if there is a specific complicated test that would solve the problem, that is the one to do (e.g. genetic testing is the best way to confirm the diagnosis of myotonic dystrophy).

Discussing management in the very limited time available is easiest if you have a mental framework to help you. Almost all management plans can be divided into:

- management of the underlying disease process
- specific symptom treatment
- general management, including long-term strategy.

Boxes 29.3 and 29.4 give some examples of how to use this approach.

BOX 29.3   ANSWERING QUESTIONS ON INVESTIGATION AND MANAGEMENT OF THE PATIENT IN BOX 29.1

Question: How would you investigate and manage this patient?

I would first review the history, in particular the speed of onset of his current problems, and seek evidence of previous neurological episodes or other significant medical problems, particularly any history of malignancy. I would ask about bladder and bowel involvement. A full examination might provide other clues, either of general medical problems or evidence of other neurological lesions. Simple investigations such as blood count, looking for anaemia, prostate-specific antigen or liver function tests and chest X-ray, as directed by the history, may be helpful, but the crucial investigation is spinal imaging to determine the nature and level of the spinal lesion. MRI is the preferred technique, which should image the spine at and above T8. This is going to determine the further investigation and management and needs to be done urgently. (*Management of the underlying disease process*). If cord compression is found, then urgent referral for neurosurgery is needed. If not, MRI of the brain, CSF examination and evoked potentials may be needed. Demyelination could be treated with steroids. (*Specific symptom management*) Pain control may be needed and bladder involvement may necessitate catheterisation. (*General management*) As the patient is immobile, prophylaxis against venous thrombosis, pressure area management and physiotherapy will all be needed. The longer-term management will depend on the cause of his spinal cord syndrome and the potential scope for recovery. Rehabilitation, including physiotherapy and occupational therapy, will be important to minimise his disability. N.B. In a younger patient, demyelination or benign tumours would be more likely; in an older patient, malignancy or degenerative changes would be more likely. Adjust your comments accordingly.

BOX 29.4 ANSWERING QUESTIONS ON INVESTIGATION AND MANAGEMENT OF THE PATIENT IN BOX 29.2

Question: How would you investigate and manage this patient?

I would first review the history, to determine the onset of the problem, any possible associated problem (for example, urinary symptoms, symptoms of postural hypotension or memory problems) and to find out how the patient is affected in everyday activities, as this will guide management. Examination might provide other useful clues; memory problems are associated with diffuse Lewy body disease, a supranuclear palsy with progressive supranuclear palsy (PSP). The diagnosis of Parkinson's disease is primarily a clinical diagnosis and further investigations are usually not needed. In younger patients, copper studies could be considered to rule out Wilson's disease. Management of Parkinson's disease is symptomatic as there is currently no treatment established to alter the underlying disease process (*management of underlying disease process*). Treatment is therefore directed at the patient's symptoms and aims to minimise his disability. Initially, milder drugs can be tried: for example, selegiline. If this patient is right-handed, it is likely that he would need to go on to the next stage, when either a dopamine agonist, such as ropinirole or pramipexole, or L-dopa, in combination with a dopa decarboxylase inhibitor, can be added, titrating the dose according to symptomatic benefit (*symptom management*). The overall strategy in the management of Parkinson's disease is to minimise the impact of the disease using as little medication as possible, to minimise adverse effects (though as much as is needed). The patient needs to understand his illness to participate in the decisions over management and thus needs to be given appropriate information. Physiotherapy and occupational therapy are helpful in maintaining function and independence. Surgery can be used later in the disease in some patients (*general management including long-term strategy*).

COMMON MISTAKES

- Failing to provide any framework for management and just listing names of drugs.
- Not considering non-medical areas of management: for example, nursing, physiotherapy and occupational therapy, or wider social issues.

LEARNING NEUROLOGICAL EXAMINATION IN A CRISIS

Hopefully very few readers will need this section, having learnt neurological examination through their training. Many students and junior doctors become anxious as they approach exams; however, they are usually a good deal more proficient than they think they are. Most can make great strides with only a little help, usually in organising their thoughts. If students get themselves into this predicament, it is often through a reluctance to practise something they feel incompetent doing.

However, sometimes people do find themselves in a fix. Proper preparation is not possible as the exam is next week. If so, this is what you need to do:

- Find one or more friends to act as examination partners to learn with you.
- Buy two (or more) copies of this book.
- Give one to each friend and read it from cover to cover (one evening).
- Practise examination of a normal subject (a willing patient or another friend), being watched by your partner, who can criticise what you are doing. Watch your partner and comment on his examination.
- Initially, practise examining by using only limited chapters, with the book to guide you. Start with elements of the examination that have a high chance of being needed in the exam:
  - *The eyes*: Chapters 7–10.
  - *Other cranial nerves*: Chapters 5, 6, 11–14.
  - *The motor system*: Chapters 4, 15–20.
  - *Limb sensation*: Chapters 21, 22.
  - *Coordination and abnormal movements*: Chapters 23, 24.
  - *Speech*: Chapter 2.
- Take it in turns to examine and to watch and advise until you are all confident with each chapter. Then practise conducting a standard examination (Chapter 28).
- Particularly practise examining the eyes (especially left eye ophthalmoscopy) and the limbs, and concentrate on developing a system of motor examination.
- Read the book again.

Having become familiar with the methods, now try to see as many patients with neurological problems as possible, again observing each other. After each examination, summarise the physical signs, come to a synthesis and differential diagnosis, and discuss the investigation and management with your examination partner, or even better with a more experienced doctor, if you can find one.

Patients are almost always keen to help. Patients with long-standing neurological problems will often be expert at being examined and are often particularly helpful.

When not seeing patients, practise describing the physical findings of imaginary patients with classical diseases and discuss their investigation and management with your examination partner.

BIBLIOGRAPHY FOR FURTHER READING AND REFERENCE

Further information about the neurological conditions mentioned in this book can be obtained in the standard textbooks listed below.

Small neurology textbooks

Fuller G, Manford M. Neurology: an illustrated colour text. 3rd edn. Churchill Livingstone: Edinburgh; 2010.

Lindsay KW, Bone I, Fuller G. Neurology and neurosurgery illustrated. 5th edn. Churchill Livingstone: Edinburgh; 2010.

Large neurology textbooks

Clarke C, Howard R, Rossor M, Shorvon SD. Neurology: a Queen Square textbook. Oxford: Wiley-Blackwell; 2009.

Ropper AH, Samuels MA. Adam and Victor's Principles of neurology. 9th edn. McGraw-Hill: New York; 2009.

Very large neurology textbooks

Daroff RB, Fenichel GM, Jankovic J, Mazziotta JC, Bradley WG. Bradley's Neurology in clinical practice. 6th edn. Butterworth-Heinemann: Boston; 2012.

Reference sources

O'Brien M. Aids to the examination of the peripheral nervous system. 5th revised edn. WB Saunders: Edinburgh; 2010.

Crossman AR, Neary D. Neuroanatomy: an illustrated colour text. 4th edn. Churchill Livingstone: Edinburgh; 2010.

General examination

Douglas G, Nichol G, Robertson C. Macleod's Clinical examination. 12th edn. Churchill Livingstone: Edinburgh; 2009.

INDEX

Note: Page numbers followed by *b* indicate boxes, *f* indicate figures and *t* indicate tables.